Lactation Management I

Edited by
Kathleen Kendall-Tackett, PhD, IBCLC, FAPA
& Scott Sherwood, BS

All royalties go to the
U.S. Lactation Consultant Association.

Praeclarus Press, LLC

Praeclarus Press, LLC

2504 Sweetgum Lane

Amarillo, Texas 79124 USA

806-367-9950

www.PraeclarusPress.com

DISCLAIMER

The information contained in this publication is advisory only and is not intended to replace sound clinical judgment or individualized patient care. The author disclaims all warranties, whether expressed or implied, including any warranty as the quality, accuracy, safety, or suitability of this information for any particular purpose.

ISBN 978-1-939807-37-3

Cover Design: Ken Tackett

Acquisition & Development: Kathleen Kendall-Tackett & Scott Sherwood

Copy Editing: Chris Tackett

Layout & Design: Nelly Murariu

Operations: Scott Sherwood

Contents

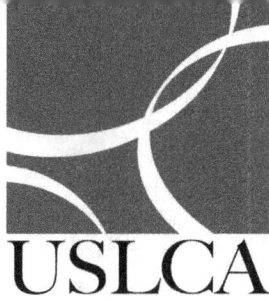

USLCA

Vitamin D

Recommendations during Pregnancy, Lactation, and Early Infancy

Carol L. Wagner, MD, FABM[1]

Keywords: pregnancy, lactation, cholecalciferol, vitamin D

Vitamin D recommendations are shifting. The Institute of Medicine recently revised the Estimated Average Requirement (EAR) from 200 to 400 international units (IU), the Recommended Dietary Allowance (RDA) from 400 to 600 international units (IU), and increased the Tolerable Upper Intake Level (UL) from 2,000 to 4,000 IU per day. What does this mean for the pregnant and lactating woman? To answer this question, current guidelines are described and adapted excerpts from a recent book on the subject are provided.

In November 2010, the Institute of Medicine (IOM) published their revised statement on vitamin D requirements (Food and Nutrition Board, 2010). Does the IOM's

1   Medical University of South Carolina, wagnercl@musc.edu

statement change how we should view vitamin D? Possibly. I believe that the IOM statement is closer to the truth. But like anything else in science, medicine, and public policy, it is a work in progress. With our current understanding, how is the IOM statement closer to the truth?

The Estimated Average Requirements (EAR), the daily amount expected to satisfy the needs of 50% of the people in that age group based on a review of the scientific literature, was increased from 200 to 400 IU/day and the Recommended Dietary Allowances (RDA; the daily dietary intake level of a nutrient considered sufficient by the Food and Nutrition Board to meet the requirements of nearly all (97–98%) healthy individuals in each life-stage and gender group) was raised to 600 IU/day (Food and Nutrition Board, 1997; 2010). The RDA is calculated based on the EAR and is usually approximately 20% higher than the EAR. Another important change made by the IOM was the increase of the Tolerable Upper Intake Levels (UL) from 2,000 to 4,000 IU/day (Food and Nutrition Board, 1997).

Are these increases adequate for the pregnant and lactating woman? In all fairness to the IOM, they had to review an inordinate amount of literature. They could not include data that had not been published. They also wanted to temper the exuberance that befalls Americans thinking that a little is good and more is better. Yet, the IOM did not extend itself to consider the overwhelming data that have emerged in the last five years that link vitamin D deficiency with immune dysfunction; rather, they restricted themselves to vitamin D and its role in maintaining bone health. As I described earlier, the IOM statement is a work in progress. With that understanding in mind, one has to reach a bit further and consider the big picture about vitamin D and how our understanding has emerged through the centuries–and it is centuries of inquiry.

Below is an excerpt and recent adaptation from the book *New Insights into Vitamin D during Pregnancy, Lactation and Early Infancy* (Wagner with Taylor & Hollis, 2010) that describes some of the issues surrounding vitamin D, as well as the current recommendations. This excerpt is meant to give you a sense of vitamin D's history and encourage you to go to the primary source for more detail.

An Overview of Vitamin D

Vitamin D is a preprohormone that has profound effects on metabolism and immune function that extend far beyond bone and calcium metabolism. We are only just beginning to understand its effects on various organ systems throughout the body—from epidemiological studies to its actions at the cellular level. Vitamin D (deficiency) has been linked to inflammatory and longlatency diseases, such as multiple sclerosis, rheumatoid arthritis, lupus, tuberculosis, diabetes, cardiovascular disease, and various cancers, to name a few. How can such a simple "vitamin" be involved in such diverse groups of diseases? What is the mechanism? What does it mean to you as an individual, practitioner, or public policy maker?

There is a renewed interest in vitamin D today. With a rise in the prevalence of vitamin D deficiency in various populations across the globe, particularly in individuals of darker pigmentation or with limited access to sunlight, there has been an urgent need to understand why this has occurred and what effect such deficiency has across the lifespan. Long-standing vitamin D deficiency is linked to a myriad of disease states through its putative effect on the immune system.

How did we get to this place of widespread vitamin D deficiency (Wagner et al., 2008)? Is vitamin D the new vitamin E and vitamin C of the 21st century, the current fad "cure-all?" Health shows, magazine articles, and the lay press write reviews trying to decipher the plethora of emerging data that is published on a weekly basis about the benefits and potential dangers of vitamin D supplementation. The individual is inundated with a vast amount of information to decipher, and to ultimately decide, "what should I do?"

For pregnant or lactating women, the question becomes even more important, as it impacts women and their unborn children, developing newborns, and infants. Health care professionals must weigh the evidence and decades-old concern that if they supplement a woman with more than 400 IU vitamin D per day, they will make her vitamin D toxic and her unborn fetus will be at risk for birth defects. Public health officials are faced with the decision of recommending higher amounts of vitamin D in vitamins and revising the national recommendations of the upper limit of what is safe for various age groups, or erring on the side of caution in maintaining the status quo because it is what has happened for the last four decades, and it is "safe." There is always the underlying tenet of "Do no harm," which must be at the heart of every recommendation. The IOM statement suggests that vitamin D deficiency is overestimated, yet using their own guidelines of a circulating 25(OH)D level of less than 20 ng/mL, in our two pregnancy studies of over 700 women, more than 75% of African American women, 50% of Hispanic women, and 20% of Caucasian women met the criteria for vitamin D deficiency (Hamilton, McNeil et al., 2010).

Dangers of Vitamin D

As early as the 1920s, reports of vitamin D toxicity surfaced. In an era when individual levels were not easily and reliably measured to document "deficiency" or "sufficiency," individuals were prescribed or given hundreds of thousands of IU's of vitamin D taken for weeks or months, which resulted in the classic symptomatology of toxicity. With careful, meticulous study, definitive "proof" of vitamin D's toxicity and teratogenicity surfaced in the early 1960s. In 1963, Black and Bonham-Carter recognized that elfin facies observed in patients with severe idiopathic infantile hypercalcemia resembled peculiar facies observed in patients with supravalvular aortic stenosis (SAS) syndrome. Shortly thereafter, Garcia et al. (1964) documented the occurrence of idiopathic hypercalcemia in an infant with SAS. The infant also had peripheral pulmonary stenosis, mental retardation, elfin facies, and an elevated blood concentration of vitamin D.

From the 1960s on, there was a rapid decline of rickets, and many believed that modern medicine and science had "cured" rickets. Unfortunately, nutritional rickets reemerged in the 1980s, particularly among African American and other darkly pigmented populations. The recurring characteristics of the reported cases were young age—particularly infants—darker pigmentation, often living at higher latitudes, and exclusive breastfeeding without vitamin D supplementation beyond 6 months of age (Rajakumar & Thomas, 2005). This finding led to a revised American Academy of Pediatrics (AAP) statement in 2003, recommending 200 IU of vitamin D supplementation to all infants receiving less than 500 ml of fortified formula per day to begin within the first 2 months of life (Gartner, Greer et al., 2003).

The question arises: If a mom's serum levels are "normal," why would you give the baby more oral vitamin D without checking the baby's serum vitamin D levels to see if more is needed? The answer is that the amount of vitamin D to achieve the lower level of normal in the mother of 32 ng/mL or 80 nmol/L (in the absence of sunlight exposure: achieved with a daily prenatal vitamin containing 400 IU up to 4,000 IU/day in some women) does not translate into adequate levels in her milk, and thus, for her baby. In this scenario, the mother is replete but on the lower end so her infant is obligated to receive 400 IU/day vitamin D to ensure adequacy in that infant. [See Wagner et al. (2006) for more information.]

Continued reports of rickets, limited dietary sources of vitamin D, inadequate sun exposure for vitamin D synthesis, and an enhanced understanding of vitamin D physiology and its actions have led to the most recent revision of the AAP statement in 2008 (Wagner, Greer, & American Academy of Pediatrics, 2008). The current recommendations are for all infants and children to be supplemented with a minimum of 400 IU per day of vitamin D, beginning in the first few days of life (Wagner, Greer et al., 2008). The issue today, however, is not too much vitamin D, but rather too little. In the past, the margin of safety of vitamin D was narrow.

There was an understandable reluctance to recommend supplementation for fear of causing toxicity. With careful study, it appears that daily vitamin D dosing of less 10,000 IU/day for extended periods is safe (Heaney et al., 2003; Vieth, 1999; Vieth & MacFarlane, 2001).

Vitamin D Recommendations for Pregnant and Lactating Women and Children

As we discussed earlier, the recommendations for vitamin D requirements have changed during the past century as the views of vitamin D's role in metabolism and toxicity have changed. It is a work in progress and each new study that helps us ascertain vitamin D's function within the body in various systems through the lifespan challenges our notion of what is required to reach optimal levels. There have been extensive data to suggest that vitamin D supplementation of 400 IU/day during the first year of life is adequate, but whether that amount is optimal remains to be proven.

Table 1. Suggested Vitamin D Supplementation Regimen for Pregnant and Lactating Women, Infants, and Children		
Age Group	Recommended Daily Vitamin D Intake (IU/day)	Caveats to Ponder
Neonates	400 IU/day	This includes premature neonates and infants. More data are needed to determine what the IU/kg requirements are of preterm infants and neonates born to mothers with frank vitamin D deficiency.
Infants < 1 year	400 IU/day up to 10 kg; then 25-50 IU/kg	
Children 1-2 yrs	25-50 IU/kg	For example, a child weighing 20 kg would be given 500-1,000 IU/day. Another child weighing 25 kg would be given 625-1,250 IU/day. One could give the lower dose during summer months and the higher dose during winter months.
Children 2-5 years	25-50 IU/kg up to 30 kg	
Children 5-12 years	25 IU/kg up to 50 kg	
Children 12-17 years	>50 kg	2,000-4,000 IU/day depending on BMI
Pregnant Women	>45 kg	4,000 IU vitamin D/day [This recommendation is based on our two RCT that were completed in 2009 (Wagner, Johnson et al., 2010; Wagner, McNeil et al., 2010).]
Lactating Women		Likely 6.400 IU/day with refinement of recommendation once Lactation RCT vitamin D studies have been completed and analyzed.

This is a conservative guide. If an individual has an increased BMI or a history of malabsorption, then that individual may require higher daily vitamin D supplementation. It would be prudent to check levels if increasing intake beyond these recommendations. The ultimate goal is to attain circulating 25(OH)D levels in that individual that would mimic living in a sun-rich environment with daily sun exposure.

The American Academy of Pediatrics (AAP) statement in 2003, recommending 200 IU of vitamin D per day, was based on the IOM's recommendation at that time centered on preventing rickets in children. Continued reports of rickets, limited dietary sources of vitamin D, inadequate sun exposure for vitamin D synthesis, and an enhanced understanding of vitamin D physiology and its actions have led to the most-recent revision of the AAP statement in 2008. The current recommendations are for all infants and children to be supplemented with a minimum of 400 IU per day of vitamin D, beginning in the first few days of life (Wagner, Greer et al., 2008). (See Chapter 9 of Wagner, with Taylor & Hollis, 2010, for further discussion on the topic.)

One size does not, nor will it ever, fit everyone. Variability in where one lives, one's diet, one's lifestyle, one's body composition (fat mass and lean body mass), and the season affect one's final vitamin D status. As the child grows, on a per kilogram basis, 400 IU/day is likely insufficient beyond a year, especially in those children with limited milk intake and sunlight exposure, in those with darker pigmentation, and who live at higher latitudes. With these caveats in mind, we can ask the question yet again: what should one do when it comes to vitamin D? The answer is found in Table 1.

Children would receive incremental doses of vitamin D based on their weight and percent body fat to maintain circulating 25(OH)D levels, with a minimum of 32 ng/ mL or 80 nmol/L (Holick, 2007; Hollis, 2005; Hollis et al., 2005; Vieth, 2009). Those children and teenagers with higher BMIs will require higher daily vitamin D intake to achieve a circulating 25(OH)D level of at least 32 ng/mL. Latitude, skin pigmentation, sunlight exposure and sunscreen use, and BMI are all factors that must be taken into account when making recommendations concerning vitamin D supplementation.

Pregnant women would be encouraged to take 4,000 IU/day[2] and lactating women at least 4,000 IU/ day, with the expected increase in the recommendation

---

2   The recommendation of 4,000 IU/day during pregnancy comes from our recently completed randomized clinical trials previously presented at Pediatric Academic Societies meeting in Vancouver, May 2010, which will be published later this year.

once studies with lactating women and their infants have been completed. Our experience thus far has been that doses of 6,400 IU/day are necessary to raise maternal milk vitamin D levels in the adequate range, so that the infant is ingesting at least 400 IU/L breastmilk. While the efficacy of this dosing regimen has been tested (Wagner et al., 2006), the safety of this regimen has not been fully tested on a large cohort of women.

On an individual basis, if a health care professional prescribes higher doses to a lactating woman, it is recommended that the woman's breastfeeding infant have levels checked to ensure that the baby is vitamin D replete. The alternative? Give the lactating woman sufficient vitamin D to achieve a total circulating 25(OH)D level of at least 80 nmol/L or 32 ng/mL and to give her breastfeeding infant the time-honored 400 IU vitamin D/day. With the latter scenario, both the mother and infant would have achieved normal vitamin D status. The downside is that both the mother and baby would need to be supplemented.

Supplementing both the lactating mother and her baby is the standard of care at this time in the U.S., with 800 IU/day recommended by the Canadians for those [adults] living above latitude 45oN (Canadian Paediatric Society, 2007). In the end, it is not sufficient to accept marginal vitamin D status, just as one would not accept or support marginal status of other hormones, such as thyroxine in someone with hypothyroidism. As is the case with every hormone, we prescribe a regimen to correct the hormonal deficiency and we do not hesitate to check a follow-up level.

The measurement of the nutritional indicator of vitamin D—namely, total circulating 25(OH)D is a fastidious and exacting process. One must ensure that the laboratory that is used has independent validation of the levels reported. Once optimal vitamin D status and how to achieve it has been determined throughout the lifespan, there will be less need to check levels. We will know through experience that 4,000 IU vitamin D/day does the trick for the pregnant woman, just as we know today that 400 IU vitamin D/day does the trick in preventing rickets and other health sequelae in young children.

Our learning curve is steep and we have come a long way since 1999 when Dr. Vieth first wowed the world with his "heretical" high-dose vitamin D safety trial (Vieth, 1999). We continue to build on the exacting rigors of scientific inquiry into the realm of vitamin D, and we should continue to demand nothing less. In the end, we must take the time to appreciate that the needs of our patients may not fit the schema that we have been taught, but rather, here before us is a challenge that will help us to better understand and redefine what is really science and medicine at its finest—discovery. It is through such discovery and positive inquiry that we will redefine the vitamin D requirements during the 21st century.

References

Black, J., & Bonham-Carter, J. (1963). Association between aortic stenosis and facies of severe infantile hypercalcemia. *Lancet, 2*, 745749.

Canadian Paediatric Society. (2007). Vitamin D supplementation: Recommendations for Canadian mothers and infants. *Paediatric & Child Health, 12*, 583-598. For full report. http://www.ncbi.nlm.nih.gov/pmc/articles/PMC2528771/?tool=pubmed

Food and Nutrition Board. Standing Committee on the Scientific Evaluation of Dietary Reference Intakes. (2010). *Dietary reference intakes for vitamin D and calcium.* Washington, D.C.: National Academy Press.

Food and Nutrition Board. Standing Committee on the Scientific Evaluation of Dietary Reference Intakes. (1997). *Dietary reference intakes for calcium, phosphorus, magnesium, vitamin D, and fluoride.* Washington, D.C.: National Academy Press.

Garcia, R.E., Friedman, W.F., Kaback, M., & Rowe, R.D. (1964). Idiopathic hypercalcemia and supravascular aortic stenosis: Documentation of a new syndrome. *New England Journal of Medicine, 271*, 117-120.

Gartner, L.M., Greer, F.R., & the American Academy of Pediatrics, Section on Breastfeeding & Committee on Nutrition. (2003). Prevention of rickets and vitamin D deficiency: New guidelines for vitamin D intake. *Pediatrics, 111*(4), 908-910.

Hamilton, S., McNeil, R., Hollis, B., et al. (2010). Profound vitamin D deficiency in a diverse group of women during pregnancy living in a sun-rich environment at latitude 32°N. *International Journal of Endocrinology*, 10.1155/2010/917428 PMCID 917428. For full report, http://www.hindawi.com/journals/ije/2010/917428.html

Heaney, R.P., Davies, K.M., Chen, T.C., Holick, M.F., & Barger-Lux, M.J. (2003). Human serum 25-hydroxycholecalciferol response to extended oral dosing with cholecalciferol. *American Journal of Clinical Nutrition, 77*, 204-210.

Hollis, B. (2005). Circulating 25-hydroxyvitamin D levels indicative of vitamin D sufficiency: Implications for establishing a new effective dietary intake recommendation for vitamin D. *Journal of Nutrition, 135*, 317-322.

Hollis, B.W., Wagner, C.L., Kratz, A., Sluss, P.M., & Lewandrowski, K.B. (2005). Normal serum vitamin D levels. Correspondence. *New England Journal of Medicine, 352,* 515-516.

Holick, M.F. (2007). Vitamin D deficiency. *New England Journal of Medicine, 357,* 266-281.

Rajakumar, K., & Thomas, S.B. (2005). Reemerging nutritional rickets: A historical perspective. *Archives of Pediatrics & Adolescent Medicine, 159*(4), 335-341.

Vieth, R. (2009). Experimentally observed vitamin D requirements are higher than extrapolated ones. *American Journal of Clinical Nutrition, 90,* 1114-1115; author reply 1115-1116.

Vieth, R. (1999). Vitamin D supplementation, 25-hydroxy-vitamin D concentrations, and safety. *American Journal of Clinical Nutrition, 69,* 842-856.

Vieth, R., Chan, P.C., & MacFarlane, G.D. (2001). Efficacy and safety of vitamin D3 intake exceeding the lowest observed adverse effect level. *American Journal of Clinical Nutrition, 73,* 288-294.

Wagner, C.L., Greer, F.R., the Section on Breastfeeding & Committee on Nutrition. (2008). Prevention of rickets and vitamin D deficiency in infants, children, and adolescents. *Pediatrics, 122,* 1142-1152.

Wagner, C.L., Hulsey, T.C., Fanning, D., Ebeling, M., & Hollis B.W. (2006). High dose vitamin D3 supplementation in a cohort of breastfeeding mothers and their infants: A six-month follow-up pilot study. *Breastfeeding Medicine, 1*(2), 59-70.

Wagner, C.L., with Taylor, S.N., & Hollis, B.W. (2010). *New insights into vitamin D during pregnancy, lactation and early infancy.* Amarillo, TX: Hale Publishing.

USLCA

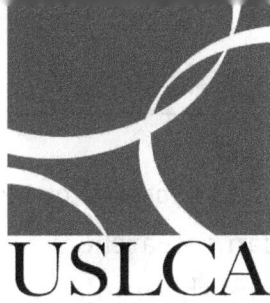

Do Recent Research Findings Mean that Mothers Should Not Take Omega-3s?

Kathleen Kendall-Tackett, PhD, IBCLC, RLC

Keywords: omega-3s, breastfeeding, depression, cognitive development

A recent study found no effect of DHA supplementation during pregnancy on maternal depression at 6 weeks and 6 months postpartum, or on babies' cognitive development. Given these results, some have been concerned about supplementing pregnant and postpartum women with omega-3s. This article examines the findings from the Makrides et al. study, and analyzes their methodology and conclusions. Based on the results of other studies, especially with regard to the omega-3 fatty acid EPA, the findings of Makrides et al. do not mean that health care providers should avoid supplementing mothers. Rather, these decisions should be based on the whole of the evidence, not a single study.

In a recent issue of the *Journal of the American Medical Association*, Australian researchers Maria Makrides and colleagues reported on the results of a large clinical trial testing the efficacy of DHA in preventing postpartum depression and increasing children's cognitive and language development at 18 months. Women were given either 800 mg of DHA or a placebo for the last half of their pregnancy. The results of their study found no significant difference in rates of depression or the baby's cognitive development in the DHA vs. placebo conditions.

In the weeks that followed publication of this article, I received several panicked emails from colleagues who were trying to understand what these findings meant. Does this mean that mothers should not take Omega-3s? But before I describe my reasons why, it might be helpful to have a small primer in Polyunsaturated Fatty Acids, known in the field as PUFAs, that will help us interpret these results.

Primer in Polyunsaturated Fatty Acids (PUFAs)

As outlined on Figure 1, PUFAs are divided into two major classes: Omega-3s and Omega-6s. Both are Essential Fatty Acids, which means that our bodies cannot manufacture them: we must consume them directly. The Omega-6s are pro-inflammatory and are found in vegetable oils. Most Americans consume these in large amounts, way more than we need, which increases our vulnerability to disease.

In contrast, Omega-3s are found in flax seed, walnuts, canola and fatty oil, coldwater fish, and are anti-inflammatory. Most Americans are deficient in these, which also makes us vulnerable to a wide range of diseases with an inflammatory etiology, including heart disease, diabetes, and depression (see Kendall-Tackett, 2007).

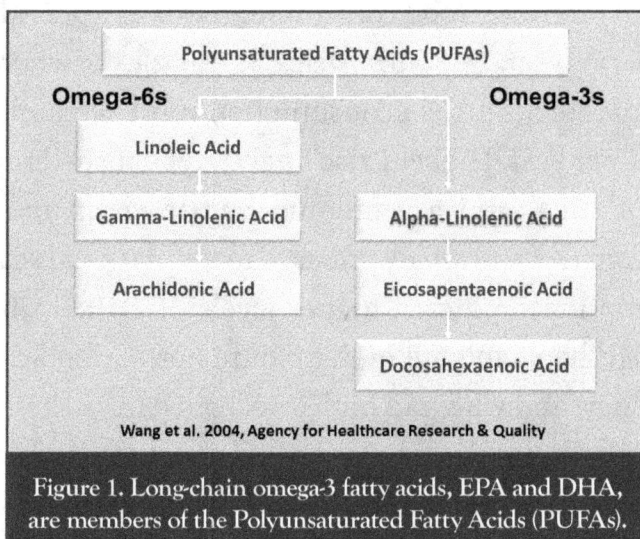

Figure 1. Long-chain omega-3 fatty acids, EPA and DHA, are members of the Polyunsaturated Fatty Acids (PUFAs).

In terms of depression, it is the long-chain Omega-3s that are of interest: EPA and DHA. These are mostly found in fish and fish-oil supplements. There is also a vegetarian source of DHA that is manufactured from algae and is an additive in infant formula and some prenatal supplements. ALA, the parent Omega-3, is found in vegetable sources, such as flax seed. Unfortunately, it is not sufficiently anti-inflammatory to be an effective treatment for depression. The majority of the studies showing that Omega-3s prevent depression are studies of fish consumption, where women are consuming both EPA and DHA (See Figure 1).

In a large cross-national ecological analysis of 41 published studies with more than 14,532 women from 22 countries, Hibbeln (2002) noted that postpartum depression was up to 50 times more common in countries with low fish consumption. For example, the rate of postpartum depression in Singapore was 0.5%, where the national rate of seafood consumption was 81.1 pounds per person, per year. In South Africa, it was 24.5%, where the national rate of seafood consumption was 8.6 pounds per person, per year. Hibbeln also analyzed published reports of DHA, EPA, and arachidonic acid levels in mothers' milk from these sample studies. Greater national seafood consumption predicted higher levels of DHA in breast milk. Mothers who ate high amounts of seafood during pregnancy, and who had high levels of DHA in their milk postpartum, had lower rates of postpartum depression. Rates of postpartum depression were not related to levels of EPA or arachidonic acid.

From the results of Hibbeln's study, it might appear as though DHA alone was key to preventing depression. But since women were consuming both EPA and DHA when they consumed fish, it's difficult to conclude that DHA alone is the effective agent. Further, studies that have examined Omega-3s as a treatment for depression have found that EPA, not DHA, is the effective component. DHA likely has a role, but the evidence has not supported it as a treatment, or even a protective agent alone. To understand why, it is helpful to examine Figure 1 again. EPA and ARA (a pro-inflammatory Omega-6) are structurally similar and compete for the same receptor sites. When EPA is not present, ARA attaches to the receptors and causes what is known as the "arachidonic cascade," leading to the release of proinflammatory cytokines, leukotrienes, eicosanoids, and prostaglandins. This explains why EPA helps a wide variety of conditions, including heart disease, metabolic syndrome, allergic/autoimmune diseases, chronic pain syndromes, and depression.

So Back to the Study Results

The methodology of the Makrides et al. study raises several concerns that limit the applicability of its findings, and to my mind do not present a compelling case against supplementing mothers with EPA and DHA.

1. They tested DHA alone as a preventative for postpartum depression. Based on what we know about why Omega-3s work for depression, the regimen should have also included EPA (EPA was included, but in an amount so small it was unlikely to have a clinical effect). Given the relative absence of EPA, I'm not at all surprised that DHA alone did not prevent depression.

2. Even if DHA could possibly have an effect by itself, the researchers discontinued it after the birth, and yet assessed depression at 6 weeks and 6 months postpartum. How was it supposed to help if mothers were not taking it postpartum?

3. The authors did not describe how the infants were fed in the first 18 months of life. That omission is huge. How many of these babies were breastfed? And for how long? And if babies were fed formula, did the formula contain added DHA? Kramer et al.'s recent clinical trial of more than 17,000 infants demonstrates that breastfeeding was related to increased cognitive development of children at age 6 (Kramer, Aboud et al. 2008). The design of the Makrides' et al. study did not control for this important contributor to infant cognitive development—namely, breastfeeding—and therefore, we must question its generalizability. Further, their design did not recognize, or control for, the role of breastfeeding in protecting maternal mental health.

4. My final point is more philosophical. DHA is being added to infant formula with promises that it boosts babies' IQ and cognitive development. There have been a number of outrageous advertisements, particularly in developing countries, showing babies using computers and wearing mortarboards. The implied promise is that this additive will produce super-smart, über-babies. The research findings on the efficacy of DHA on cognitive development have been far more mixed, or even negative [see recent Cochrane review]. Unfortunately, the design of the Makrides et al. study was influenced by this fairly simplistic and mechanistic model of cognitive development: add a substance, boost IQ.

5. In reality, cognitive development is influenced by a wide range of factors, including mother-baby interaction—and breastfeeding. It's not simply a matter of adding a substance to the milk that babies consume. It is also important to point out that all of the authors on this study have been funded by and/or serve as advisors for formula companies, including Nestle, Fonterra, and Nutricia. The authors were careful to disclose their affiliations with formula companies, and their funders were not involved in the research design or analysis of results. Nevertheless, the researchers have served as advisors to companies making infant formulas with DHA. It would be difficult for them not to be influenced by the model that guides much of the research into infant formulas with added DHA (i.e., that simply adding DHA will have these profound effects).

The Bottom Line

I do not believe that the Makrides et al. study indicates that mothers should not be supplemented with Omega-3s, as most women are deficient in these, and supplementing will likely improve their overall physical and mental well-being [see Kendall-Tackett, 2010 for more information]. But supplements should include both EPA and DHA (at least 800 mg of each). We should continue to support breastfeeding, as it both aides in babies' cognitive development and lowers women's risk for depression.

References

Hibbeln, J. R. (2002). Seafood consumption, the DHA content of mothers' milk and prevalence rates of postpartum depression: A cross-national, ecological analysis. *Journal of Affective Disorders, 69*, 15-29.

Kramer, M. S., F. Aboud, et al. (2008). Breastfeeding and child cognitive development. *Archives of General Psychiatry, 65*(5), 578584.

Kendall-Tackett, K. A. (2007). A new paradigm for depression in new mothers: The central role of inflammation and how breastfeeding and anti-inflammatory treatments protect maternal mental health. *International Breastfeeding Journal,* 2:6. doi:doi:10.1186/1746-4358-2-6.

Kendall-Tackett, K. A. (2010). Long-chain omega-3 fatty acids and women's mental health in the perinatal period. *Journal of Midwifery and Women's Health, 55*(6), 561-567.

Makrides, M., Gibson, R. A., McPhee, A. J., Yelland, L., Quinlivan, J., Ryan, P., & DOMInO Investigative Team. (2010). Effect of DHA supplementation during pregnancy on maternal depression and neurodevelopment of young children. *JAMA, 304*(15), 1675-1683.

This article is being re-published with permission from Lamaze International. First publication appeared as a blog post at http:// www.scienceandsensibility.com on December 6, 2010.

USLCA

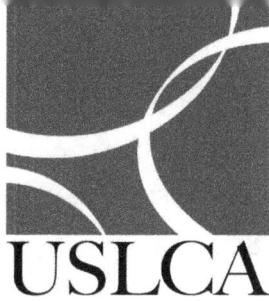

Breastfeeding and the Use of Contrast Dyes for Maternal Tests

Kay Hoover, M. Ed., IBCLC, RLC, FILCA

Keywords: breastfeeding, contrast dyes, X-rays

The current recommendation from the American College of Radiology concerning iodinated X-ray contrast media (ionic and non-ionic) and gadolinium-based contrast agents states:

> ... we believe that the available data suggest that it is safe for the mother and infant to continue breastfeeding after receiving such an agent.

Frustrated with the mixed messages our postpartum families were receiving, I developed a poster on contrast dyes to help our hospital nurses and the radiology department, with the assistance of Dr. Tom Hale, members of the Pennsylvania Resource Organization for Lactation

Consultants, Barbara Wilson-Clay, Donna Butler, Cindy Griffis, and Jeanne Spencer.

I list the 21 dyes that are available in the U.S. on the back of the poster, based on the listings in Medications and Mothers' Milk (Hale, 2010). This listing was reviewed on several occasions by both Dr. Hale and my local chapter of USLCA. Please feel free to copy and distribute this poster widely. Click here for the full-page version of the poster and list of contrast agents. I am happy to email the front and back sides of the poster so you have it in a Word document. Contact me at kay@hoover.net

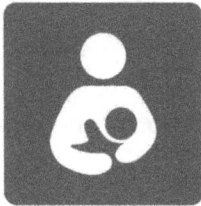

It is safe
to breastfeed right after a scan with a contrast dye

Except for Teslascan (Mangafodipir Trisodium)

Radiocontrast Agents and Breastfeeding

Safe Radiocontrast Agents

Barium Sulfate

Not absorbed orally, none will enter the milk
No interruption in breastfeeding is necessary[2]

Bilopaque (Tyropanoate)

Oral contrast agent for examining the gallbladder
Levels in milk are unknown[2]

Gadolinium-Containing Radiocontrast Agents

"Review of the literature shows no evidence to suggest that oral ingestion by an infant of the tiny amount of gadolinium contrast agent excreted into breast milk would cause toxic effects. We believe, therefore, that the available data suggest that it is safe for the mother and infant to continue breastfeeding after receiving such an agent."[1]

Magnevist (Gadopentetate)	Omniscan (Gadodiamide)
Magnevistan (Gadopentetate)	Optimark (Gadoversetamide)
Magnograf (Gadopentetate)	Prohance (Gadoteridol)
MultiHance (Gadobenate)	Viewgam (Gadopentetate)

Iodinated containing radiopaque medium (Ionic and Nonionic)

"Because of the very small percentage of iodinated contrast medium that is excreted into the breast milk and absorbed by the infant's gut, we believe that the available data suggest that it is safe for the mother and infant to continue breastfeeding after receiving such an agent."[1]

Accupaque (Iohexol)	Gastromiro (Iopamidol)	Optiray (Ioversol)
Amipaque (Metrizamide)	Gastrovist (Diatrizoate)	Pamiray (Iopamidol)
Angio-Conray (Iothalamate)	Hexabrix 160 (Ioxaglate)	Proscope (Iopromide)
Angiocontrast (Metrizoate)	Hexabrix 200 (Ioxaglate)	Radiomiron (Iopamidol)
Angiovist (Diatrizoate)	Hexabrix 320 (Ioxaglate)	Reno-30 (Diatrizoate)
Biliopaco (Iopromide)	Hexabrix (Ioxaglate)	Reno-60 (Diatrizoate)
Cardiografin (Diatrizoate)	Hypaque (Diatrizoate)	Reno-Dip (Diatrizoate)
Cholografin (Iodipamide)	Isopaque (Metrizoate)	Renografin (Diatrizoate)
Cistobil (Iopromide)	Iopamiro (Iopamidol)	Reno-M (Diatrizoate)
Clarograf (Iopromide)	Iopamiron (Iopamidol)	Retrografin (Diatrizoate)
Colegraf (Iopromide)	Iopasen (Iopamidol)	Scanlux (Iopamidol)
Colepak (Iopromide)	Isovue (Iopamidol)	Sinografin (Diatrizoate)
Conray-30 (Iothalamate)	Isovue-M (Iopamidol)	Sinografin (Iodipamide)
Conray-43 (Iothalamate)	Jopamiro (Iopamidol)	Solutrast (Iopamidol)
Conray-60 (Iothalamate)	Myelo-Kit (Iohexol)	Telebrix (Ioxitalamic Acid)
Conray 325 (Iothalamate)	Neocontrast (Iopromide)	Telepaque (Iopanoic Acid)
Conray-400, (Iothalamate)	Niopam (Iopamidol)	Ultravist (Iopromide)
Cyso-Conray (Iothalamate)	Omnigraf (Iohexol)	Urovist (Diatrizoate)
Cysto-Conray II (Iothalamate)	Omnipaque (Iohexol)	Vascoray (Iothalamate)
Cystografin (Diatrizoate)	Omnitrast (Iohexol)	Visipaque (Iodixanol)
Ethibloc (Diatrizoate)	Optiject (Ioversol)	

Radiocontrast Agent of Concern

Teslascan (Mangafodipir Trisodium)

Manganese-containing radiocontrast agent	A brief interruption of breastfeeding for 4 hours
Rapidly redistributed to liver	followed by pumping and dumping her milk once
Save milk ahead of the test for one or two feedings	This would reduce any risk to the infant[2]

Bibliography

[1]American College of Radiology, Committee on Drugs and Contrast Media (2010). *Administration of contrast media to breastfeeding mothers*, ACR Manual on Contrast Media, Version 7.
[2]Hale T. (2010). *Medications and mothers' milk* (14th Ed). Amarillo, TX: Hale Publishing. pp. 1150-1151, 1153
Infant-Risk Center—Call to check if medications compatible with breastfeeding (Monday-Friday 9 am to 6 pm EST, 806-352-2519.)

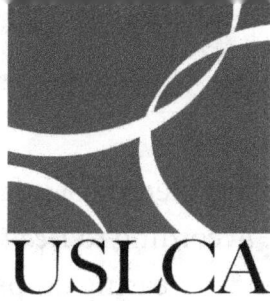

Marijuana Use and Breastfeeding

Carrie W. Miller, MSN, RN, CNE, IBCLC, RLC[1]

Keywords: breastfeeding, marijuana, substance abuse, mothering, infants

Marijuana is one of the most widely used recreational substances in the United States, with high rates of use during peak childbearing years. Medical marijuana use is also becoming more widely accepted in the United States, with legalization in 17 states and the District of Columbia. The available literature suggests that maternal marijuana use during breastfeeding is associated with potentially negative outcomes for infants and children. Adverse effects can include feeding difficulty, lethargy, and delayed cognitive and motor development. Mothers considered heavy or chronic users of marijuana are advised to not breastfeed infants. The aim of this article is to examine the prevalence of marijuana use, the potential effects on breastfed infants, and current recommendations from lactation experts.

---

1   millerca@seattleu.edu, Washington State University, College of Nursing, Spokane, Washington. There are no conflicts of interest to disclose.

Breastfeeding is the best method of infant nutrition during the first year of life. According to *Healthy People 2020*, new objectives recommend increasing the percentage of infants "ever" breastfed from 75% to 81.9%. Human milk provides superior nutritional and health opportunities, optimizing both maternal and infant health. However, an infant exposed to maternal use of marijuana prenatally or after birth may present with feeding difficulties, withdrawal symptoms, and growth delays (deDios, et al., 2010; Garry et al., 2009; Simmons et al., 2009). Marijuana is a widely used recreational substance in the United States, with the highest rates of use between ages 18 to 25, and greatest increases in use seen in childbearing women (deDios, et al., 2010; Garry et al., 2009). Studies conducted in Europe and the United States from 1980 to 2000 suggest rates between 3% to 30%, with average rates between 10% to 15% (Garry et al., 2009). According to the National Survey on Drug Use and Health, 15.2 million people have used illicit drugs in the past 30 days, with 53.3% of users citing marijuana as the drug of choice (National Institutes on Drug Abuse [NIDA], 2011).

Marijuana grows naturally in most parts of the world and is legal for medicinal uses in 17 of the United States and the District of Columbia. The active ingredient in marijuana is delta-9-tetrahydrocannabinol (THC), which is responsible for the desired effects (NIDA, 2010) (See Table 1). Accepted medical diagnoses for medical marijuana use include analgesia for acute and chronic pain, migraine, post-traumatic stress, cachexia, nausea, tremor, anxiety, and epilepsy (Garry et al., 2009; Kurtz et al., 2010).

Table 1. Effects of Marijuana Use

Desired Effects	Adverse Effects
• Euphoria	• Panic attacks
• Increased appetite	• Impaired use of motor vehicle
• Altered perception	• Dizziness
• Sedation	• Altered perception
• Decreased pain	• Possible reduction in prolactin levels
• Reduced anxiety	• Increased heart rate
• Increased sense of confidence	• Delayed response time

Maternal marijuana use during pregnancy and lactation is associated with potentially negative outcomes for infants and children. Hale and Hartman (2006) report using marijuana during lactation can affect brain development of the growing infant. However, as more states legalize medical marijuana, childbearing women need to be advised of the benefits of breastfeeding and the potential negative outcomes of using marijuana while breastfeeding (Garry et al., 2009; Hale & Hartman, 2006; Morrison et al., 2010). Lactation consultants, nurses, and medical providers need to recognize the specialized care of these maternal/infant dyads to promote healthy outcomes. This article examines the prevalence of marijuana use in childbearing and breastfeeding women, the potential effects to infants, and current recommendations for lactation consultants.

Health Promotion

Under most circumstances, human beings strive to maintain or improve their health. Health-promoting activities can vary based on societal and cultural expectations and how one achieves ideal health in the face of chronic disease (Pender et al., 2011; Sheehan et al., 2010). Individuals using medicinal marijuana to decrease symptoms of chronic illness are striving for health promotion. To have less pain, anxiety, tremor, nausea, post-traumatic stress, and cachexia related to cancer, hepatitis C, or AIDS are powerful attractants to reduce symptoms affecting quality of life. Breastfeeding is another health-promoting activity (AAP, 2012; Healthy People 2020; WHO, 2012). In 2011, Surgeon General Benjamin issued a statement encouraging women to breastfeed as the best way to nourish infants and protect them from disease (Dewey et al., 2003; Hale & Hartman, 2006; Lawrence & Lawrence, 2005).

Legalized Marijuana in the United States

In the United States, marijuana is still considered a Schedule I drug [high potential for abuse] by the U.S. Drug Enforcement Agency. The possible medicinal effects of marijuana have been the subject of research and debate. Legislative support for legalizing medical marijuana was established under the Compassionate Use Act in 1996 by California Health and Safety Code, Proposition 215 (Office of National Drug Policy [ONDCP], 2003). In several states, patients are allowed to have multiple plants and up to 8 ounces of usable marijuana in their possession (Kurtz et al., 2010).

Medicinal marijuana is obtained through medical marijuana distributors. Currently in the United States, 17 states and District of Columbia allow legalized use of medical marijuana with a prescription for several chronic conditions to improve quality of life (see Table 2). Medical providers are required to perform a physical examination and health assessment to determine eligibility for medicinal marijuana, with each state offering specific guidelines. Approved conditions may include cancer, cachexia, epilepsy, glaucoma, chronic severe pain, migraine, or nausea (Kurtz et al., 2010). Less common uses include insomnia, attention deficit hyperactivity disorder (ADHD), post-traumatic stress disorder (PTSD), and anxiety (Garry et al., 2009; Kurtz et al., 2010).

Table 2. States with Legalized Marijuana

	Year Passed		Year Passed
Alaska	1998	Michigan	2008
Arizona	2010	Montana	2004
California	1996	Nevada	2000
Colorado	2000	New Jersey	2010
Connecticut	2012	New Mexico	2007
District of Columbia (DC)	2010	Oregon	1998
Delaware	2011	Rhode Island	2006
Hawaii	2000	Vermont	2004
Maine	1999	Washington	1998

Reference: www.Procon.org

The Mechanisms and Effects of Marijuana Use

Marijuana is traditionally inhaled using glassware pipes or hand rolled in the form of a cigarette. Once inhaled, marijuana reaches peak effect within 10 minutes, with an expected duration of two to three hours. In marijuana smoke, more than 400 compounds are present with the main hallucinogenic ingredient: delta-9-Tetra-Hydro-Cannabinol (Djulus et al., 2005; Hale & Hartman, 2006; NIDA, 2011). THC is the "agonist of the cannabinoid receptors located in the nervous system" (Garry et a.l, 2009, p. 2). Cannabinoid receptors (CB) are found in high quantities in specific areas of the brain, including areas influencing thought, concentration, memory, pleasure, perception of time and pain, and finally, cognitive concentration (NIDA, 2010). Cannabinoid receptors also act on brain development during fetal life and play a critical role after birth in the initiation of infant suckling (Garry et al., 2009). The effects of THC manifests on the mesocorticolimbic system and can inhibit gammaaminobutyric acid (GABA) release, resulting in lack of inhibition of dopamiergic neurons (deDios et al., 2010; Garry et al., 2009).

Desired effects for marijuana users include pain relief, altered perception, sedation, euphoria, relaxation, altered mood, delayed response, increased hunger signals, and sense of calm (see Table 1), (deDios et al., 2010; Garry et al., 2009; Hale & Hartman, 2006; Sheih & Kravitz, 2006). Adverse effects include muscle weakness, anxiety,

37

panic attacks, increased heart rate, and increased risk of depressive symptoms in adults (Garry et al., 2009; Hale, 2010). Additional adverse effects from marijuana inhalation or ingestion include poor short-term memory, impaired motor performance, and dizziness (Djulus et al., 2005; Hale & Hartmann, 2006).

Marijuana also can be added to food products, oil infusions, and butters (Chapkis & Webb, 2005). Ingestion of marijuana can take up to an hour to peak, with effects lasting several hours (Chapkis & Webb, 2005). The half-life of THC for an adult is one to 2.3 days and it is metabolized through the kidneys (Hale, 2010). Urine testing for four to six weeks post-inhalation or ingestion is an effective way to determine use in the adult population (Day et al., 2006; Garry et al., 2009; Hansen et al., 2008; Shieh & Kravitz, 2006; Williams & Ross, 2007).

Prevalence of Marijuana Use

Rates of recreational marijuana use are increasing. According to deDios et al. (2010), young adults ages 18 to 25 have the highest rate of marijuana use, with 16.4% reporting use within the past month. Five percent of childbearing women, ages 15 to 44 years, reported using marijuana in the past 30 days, according to National Survey on Drug Use and Health (Substance Abuse and Mental Health Services Administration, 2007). Garry et al. (2009) reported that marijuana is the most commonly used recreational drug used during pregnancy, with rates ranging from 3% to 30% percent in studies conducted in

Europe and the United States. Recent national estimates in the United States suggest 9.8% of all women, ages 15 to 44 years, and 4% of pregnant women report using illicit drugs in the past month, with marijuana being the most commonly used (Schempf & Strobino, 2008).

According to deDios et al. (2010), complications from the use in young women, ages 18 to 29, have increased from 25% in the 1990s to 32% in 2002. Adverse effects can include increased risky sexual activity, polysubstance abuse, and poor judgment regarding parenting (deDios et al., 2010; Garry et al., 2009; Shieh & Kravitz, 2006). There are no known studies describing the rates of medicinal marijuana use in breastfeeding women. The challenge may be that childbearing women are reluctant to report marijuana use because they are afraid of legal consequences and possible interference by child protective services (Garry et al., 2009; Simmons et al., 2009).

Breastfeeding and Marijuana Use

The benefits of human milk are well known. However, when marijuana is inhaled or ingested by a lactating woman, THC crosses over into the breast milk and can be absorbed by the nursing infant (Academy of Breastfeeding Medicine [ABM], 2009; Astley & Little, 1990; Garry et al., 2009; Perez-Reyes & Wall, 1982). Breastfed infants exposed to THC in the first months of life will metabolize and absorb marijuana compounds at a time when brain development is rapid (Garry et al., 2009). An infant will test positive for marijuana in urine for two to three weeks after ingesting breast milk that contains THC (Garry et al., 2009; Liston, 1998). Infants exposed to THC through breast milk are reported to have increased tremors, poor sucking, slow weight gain, and poor feeding in the first month of life (see Table 3) (Astley & Little, 1990; Garry et al., 2009).

Table 3. Adverse Effects on Breastfeeding Infants
• Increased tremor
• Poor sucking reflex
• Decreased feeding time
• Slow weight gain
• Changes in visual responses
• Delayed motor development

Studies in animals suggest prolactin levels may be reduced with marijuana use and may inhibit milk supply. However, this has not been proven in human populations (Garry et al., 2009; Hale & Hartmann, 2006). With reduction in prolactin levels, milk production may be reduced for the growing infant and can impede normal growth and development (Dewey et al., 2003; Garry et al., 2009; Rasmussen & Kjolhede, 2004). Based on available evidence, infants fed human milk containing marijuana may gain weight more slowly, have ineffective sucking patterns, be at risk for failure to thrive, and have increased risk for sudden infant death syndrome (SIDS) (Astley & Little, 1990; Djulus et al., 2005; Garry et al., 2009).

Fried (1980) studied neonates exposed prenatally to THC and concluded infants of heavy marijuana users were more likely to have a heightened startle reflex and increased jitteriness, consistent with drug withdrawal. A Letter to the Editor in the *New England Journal of Medicine* presented a case study of two breastfeeding mothers: one mother smoked marijuana once a day and the second mother smoked seven times daily (Perez-Reyes & Wall, 1982). Breast milk was analyzed one-hour post inhalation. The breast milk from the mother who smoked seven times a day had TCH levels eight times higher than in her blood levels. Fecal analysis of the infant showed positive metabolites in the baby's stools, suggesting THC in breast milk was metabolized by the infant (Perez-Reyes & Wall, 1982). The mother who smoked only once daily, THC was considered nominal in mother's milk and the infant's urine screen was negative (Pérez-Reyes & Wall, 1982). Limitations of the case study include lack of consistency of amount of time between inhalation of marijuana and infant exposure, and the small sample size.

In 1985, Tennes et al. followed 62 infants in the first year of life. Of the study group, 27 of the mothers reported using marijuana during breastfeeding: 12 smoked once a month or less, nine weekly, and six daily. The results suggested no significant differences in adverse events between the babies of the non-users vs. users of marijuana exposed through breast milk (Tennes et al., 1985). Astley and Little (1990) suggested that infants exposed to marijuana via breast milk were more likely to exhibit adverse effects of THC at one month than they were at three months and one year. Fried and Watkinson (1990) investigated verbal and memory domains in 4-year-old children exposed to marijuana prenatally and after birth. At 4 years, children exposed to maternal marijuana had significantly lower scores in memory and verbal domains.

Studies have shown marijuana can adversely affect infants; however, the evidence is conflicting. Therefore, results need to be considered cautiously when regarding sample size, maternal self-reporting integrity, and study type. Another issue may be the differences in potency of plants, levels of THC, or methods of measurements. According to the Office of National Drug Control Policy (2003), marijuana plants today have more THC, with a six-fold increase in potency than plants available 30 years ago.

Another consideration is the ethical challenges of researching women breastfeeding using marijuana. Researchers report potential harm to the mother and infant when using marijuana, creating conflict of human protection in health research studies (Djulus et al., 2005; Garry et al., 2009; Sheih & Kravitz, 2006; Simmons et al., 2009). The primary challenge faced by lactation counselors and medical providers is the lack of consistent, current, and evidence-based research for this population (ABM, 2009).

Implications for Practice

According to the Academy of Breastfeeding Medicine (2009), providing support for a mother who wants to breastfeed and use marijuana, either recreationally or medicinally, is challenging. Infants can be at risk for multiple difficulties, both physically and developmentally. However, they can benefit from human milk and breastfeeding. The Academy of Breastfeeding Medicine and International Lactation Consultant Association (ILCA) encourage medical providers and lactation consultants to prepare pregnant women for lactation and postpartum marijuana abstinence to promote advantageous outcomes (ABM, 2009; ILCA, 2009).

The Academy of Breastfeeding Medicine (2009), Hale (2010), and the American Academy of Pediatrics (2012) recommend that women avoid breastfeeding if they consistently or heavily use marijuana, either recreationally or medicinally. Further, women who do not receive consistent prenatal care, have a positive urine drug screen at time of delivery, and have no confirmed plan of care at the time of delivery should not breastfeed. When breastfeeding is contraindicated, mothers need information regarding banked human milk and preparation of artificial baby milk. The rationale for this recommendation is clear; the available evidence suggests that THC passes through the breast milk and can potentially adversely affect the breastfed infant (ABM, 2009; Astley & Little, 1990; Garry et al., 2009; Hale, 2010).

Mothers need to be educated to the potential adverse effects related to feeding challenges, delayed growth, and development. Further education for mothers consists of discouraging smoking marijuana around the infant or within the home setting to reduce exposure of second-hand smoke (Garry et al., 2009). Lactation consultants working with mothers who occasionally use medicinal marijuana require careful consideration and education regarding the half-life of THC, amount of exposure to the infant, and follow-up care. Careful observation of the mother and infant, while maintaining an open and trusting relationship with the maternal-infant dyad, will ensure opportunities for education and informed decision making. There are no studies that support breastfeeding and use of marijuana. However, with conflicting results, further studies and case-by-case considerations are warranted in cases of occasional use.

Conclusion

Medical marijuana is known to offer improvement for symptoms of chronic illness and these benefits have been recognized by voters, state legislation, and medical providers. Conditions, such as pain, ADHD, depression, anxiety, nausea, and post-traumatic stress disorder are possible diagnoses for which medical marijuana may be prescribed. The challenge faced by medical providers and lactation consultants is the limited studies with conflicting research results about whether limited use is harmful. Current evidence-based support is lacking in regard to these recommendations. Guidelines through the Academy of Breastfeeding Medicine and International Lactation Consultant Association have clearly identified the value of breast milk, and many medications and substances are considered acceptable for women to use during breastfeeding. However, recreational or medical marijuana use is more of a cause for concern and requires individualized assessment, plan of care, and follow-up. Lactation consultants, medical providers, and peer counselors need to carefully consider how to advise women who choose to use marijuana and still offer the best nutrition to their infants.

References

Academy of Breastfeeding Medicine Protocol Committee. (2009). ABM Clinical protocol #21: Guidelines for breastfeeding and the drug dependent woman. *Breastfeeding Medicine, 4*, 225-228. Doi: 10.1089/bfm.2009.9987

American Academy of Pediatrics (2004). Legalization of marijuana: Potential impact on youth. *Pediatrics, 113*, 1825. Retrieved from http://pediatrics.aappublications.org/content/113/6/1825.full.pdf+html

American Academy of Pediatrics (2001). Committee on drugs. The transfer of drugs and other chemicals into human milk. *Pediatrics, 108*, 766-789. Retrieved from http://pediatrics.aappublications.org/content/108/3/776.full.pdf+html

American Academy of Pediatrics (2012). Breastfeeding and use of human milk: Section on Breastfeeding. *Pediatrics, 129*, e827. Doi: 10.1542/peds.2011-3552. Retrieved from http://pediatrics.aappublications.org/content/129/3/e827

Astley, S., & Little, R. (1990). Maternal marijuana use during lactation and infant development at one year. *Neurotoxicology and Teratology, 12*, 161-168.

Chapkis, W., & Webb, R. (2005). Mother's milk and the muffin man: Grassroots innovations in medical marijuana delivery systems. *Journal of Ethnicity in Substance Abuse, 4*(3/4), 183-204. Doi: 10.1300/J233v04n03_08

Day, N., Goldschmidt, L., & Thomas, C. (2006). Prenatal marijuana exposure contributes to the prediction of marijuana use at age 14. *Addiction, 101,* 1313-1322. Doi: 10.1111/j.13600443.2006.01523.x

deDios, M., Hagerty, C., Herman, D., Hayaki, J., Anderson, B., Budney, A., & Stein, M. (2010). General anxiety disorder symptoms, tension reduction, and marijuana use among young adult females. *Journal of Women Health, 19,* 1635-1642. Doi: 10.1089/jwh.2010.1973

Dewey, K., Nommsen-Rivers, L., Heinig, M., & Cohen, R. (2003). Risk factors for suboptimal infant feeding behavior, delayed onset of lactation, and excess neonatal weight loss. *Pediatrics, 112,* 607-619.

Djulus, J., Moretti, M., & Koren, G. (2005). Marijuana use and breastfeeding. Canadian Family Physician, 51, 349-350. Fried, P. (1980). Marijuana use by pregnant women: Neurobehavioral effects in neonates. *Drug and Alcohol Dependence, 6,* 415-424.

Fried, P., & Watkinson, B. (1990). 36 and 48 month neurobehavioral follow-up of children prenatally exposed to marijuana, cigarettes, and alcohol. *Journal of Development & Behavioral Pediatrics, 11*(2), 49-58. Doi: 10.1097/00004703199004000-00003

Garry, A., Rigourd, V., Amirouche, A., Fauroux, V., Aubry, S., & Serreau, R. (2009). Cannibis and breastfeeding. *Journal of Toxicology.* Doi: 10.1155/2009/596149

Hale, T., & Hartman, P. (2006). *Textbook of human lactation.* Amarillo, Texas: Hale Publishing.

Hale, T. (2010). *Medications and mothers' milk, 14th ed..* Amarillo, Texas: Hale Publishing.

Hansen, H.H., Krutz, B., & Sifringer, M., et al. (2008). Cannabinoids enhance susceptibility of immature brain to ethanol neurotoxicity. *Annals of Neurology, 64,* 42-52. Doi: 10.1002/ana.21287.

Healthy People 2020. (2012). *Increase the proportion of infant who are breastfed. Maternal, infant and child health. U.S. Department of Health and Human Services.* Retrieved from http://healthypeople. gov/2020/topicsobjectives2020/ebr. aspx?topicId=26

International Lactation Consultant Association. (2009). *Standards of practice for international board certified lactation consultants.* Retrieved from http://www.ilca.org/files/resources/ Standards-of-Practice-web.pdf

Kurtz, J., Markoff, J., McNall, B., & Shimohara, S. (2011). *16 legal marijuana states and DC.* Retrieved from www.Procon.org

Lawrence, R., & Lawrence, R. (2005). *Breastfeeding: A guide for the medical profession.* Philadelphia: Elsevier Mosby.

Liston, J. (1998). Breastfeeding and the use of recreational drugsalcohol, caffeine, nicotine and marijuana. *Breastfeeding Review, 6*(2), 27-30.

Morrison, D., Lohr, M., Beadnell, B., Gillmore, M., Lewis, S., & Gilchrist, M. (2010). Young mothers decisions to use marijuana: A test of an expanded theory of planned behavior. *Psychology and Health, 25,* 569-587. Doi: 10.1080/08870440902777554

National Institute on Drug Abuse. (2010). *Research report series: Marijuana abuse.* Retrieved from http://www.drugabuse.gov/ publications/research-reports/marijuana-abuse

National Institute on Drug Abuse. (2011). *Topics in brief: Marijuana.* Retrieved from http://www.drugabuse.gov/drugsabuse/marijuana

Office of National Drug Control Policy. (2003). *What Americans need to know about marijuana. Annual Report, ONDCP.* Retrieved from www.whitehouse.gov/ondcp

Office of the Surgeon General. (2011). *Surgeon General's Call to Action to Support Breastfeeding.* Retrieved from http://www. surgeongeneral.gov/topics/breastfeeding/factsheet.html

Pender, N., Murdaugh, C., & Parsons, M. (2011). *Health promotion in nursing practice.* Upper Saddle River: New Jersey: Pearson.

Perez-Reyes, M., & Wall, M. (1982). Presence of delta-9tetrahydrocannabinol in human milk. *New England Journal of Medicine, 307*(13), 819-820.

Rasmussen, K., & Kjolhede, C. (2004). Prepregnant overweight and obesity diminish the prolactin response to suckling in the first week postpartum. *Pediatrics, 113*, 465-471.

Schempf, A., & Strobino, D. (2008). Illicit drug use and adverse birth outcomes: Is it drugs or context? *Journal of Urban Health: Bulletin of the New York Academy of Medicine, 85*(6), 858-873. Doi: 10.1007/s11524-008-9315-6

Sheehan, A., Schmied, V., & Barclay, L. (2010). Complex decisions: Theorizing women's infant feeding decisions in the first 6 weeks after birth. *Journal of Advanced Nursing, 66*, 371-380. Doi: 10.1111/j.1365-2648.2009.05194.x

Shieh, C., & Kravitz, M. (2006). Severity of drug use, initiation of prenatal care, and maternal-fetal attachment in pregnant marijuana and cocaine/heroin users. *Journal of Women's Health, Obstetrics and Neonatal Nurses, 35*, 499-508. Doi: 10.1111/J.15526909.2006.00063.x

Simmons, L., Havens, J., Whiting, J., Holz, J., & Bada, H. (2009). Illicit drug use among women with children in the United States 2002-2003. *Annuals of Epidemiology, 19*, 187-193. Doi: 10.1016/j.annepidem.2008.12.007

Substance Abuse and Mental Health Services Administration. (2007). *Results from the 2006 National Survey on Drug Use and Health: National findings* (Office of Applied Studies, NSDUH Series H-32, DHHS Publication No. SMA 07-4293). Rockville, MD. Retrieved from http://www.samhsa.gov/data/nsduh/2k6nsduh/2k6results.pdf

Tennes, K., Avitable, N., Blackard, C., Boyles, C., Hassoun, B., Holmes, L., & Kreye, M. (1985). *Marijuana: Prenatal and postnatal exposure in the human.* National Institute on Drug Abuse, 59, 48-60.

Williams, J., & Ross, L. (2007). Consequences of prenatal toxin exposure for mental health in children and adolescents. *European Child & Adolescent Psychiatry, 16*, 243-253. Doi: 10.1007/s00787-006-0596-6

World Health Organization. (2012). *Health topics: Breastfeeding.* Retrieved from http://www.who.int/topics/breastfeeding/en/

For the past 21 years, **Carrie Miller** has explored multiple areas of nursing, including maternal/child, lactation, operating room, sexual assault nurse examiner, and nursing education. Her primary focus is maternal/child and lactation consulting. She received her undergraduate degree in nursing from Oregon Health Sciences University in 1991, Masters in Nursing Education from University of Phoenix in 2006, and is actively pursuing a PhD in nursing research at Washington State University. She is currently working as an instructor at Seattle University in Seattle Washington.

The Affordable Care Act Provides Benefits for Expectant Mothers and Their Newborns

The Affordable Care Act helps make prevention affordable and accessible for all Americans by requiring health plans to cover recommended preventive services without cost sharing. Starting August 2012, the Department of Health and Human Services (HHS) adopted additional Guidelines for Women's Preventive Services that will be covered without cost sharing. These include support for breastfeeding; well-woman visits; screening for gestational diabetes, HIV, and sexually transmitted infections; contraception; and domestic violence screening.

Pregnant and postpartum women will have access to comprehensive lactation support and counseling from trained providers, as well as breastfeeding equipment. One of the barriers for breastfeeding is the cost of purchasing or renting breast pumps and related supplies. The guidelines were based on scientific evidence and were recommended by the independent Institute of Medicine (IOM). To learn more about preventive services for women, visit Healthcare.gov.

Three Midwifery Organizations Issue Consensus Statement

The United States' three midwifery organizations, American College of Nurse-Midwives, Midwives Alliance of North America (MANA), and National Association of Certified Professional Midwives (NACPM), released a historic consensus statement. *Supporting Healthy and Normal Physiologic Childbirth: A Consensus Statement* gives maternity care providers, policymakers, and women a succinct summary of the evidence for the benefits of normal physiologic childbirth.

USLCA

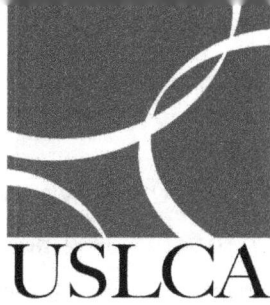

Parenting Plans and the Breastfed Child

A Look at How Breastfeeding is Used as a Factor in Parenting Time Allocations for Divorcing Parents in the U.S.

Kori Martin, JD, LLLL

Keywords: parenting plans, custody, breastfeeding, divorce

Divorce has the potential to substantially disrupt a mother and baby's breastfeeding relationship, due to the potential for separation inherent in custody and visitation schedules. This paper examines how breastfeeding is accounted for as a factor in the parenting plan guidelines actually used in the United States legal system. While some jurisdictions do include breastfeeding as a specific factor to be included in the allocation of parenting time, most courts have no legislative or rule-based guidance as to how breastfeeding should be accounted for post-divorce. The breastfeeding protections that do exist get noticeably more restrictive as the child ages, and mothers in the U.S. currently face significant hurdles in preserving breastfeeding post-divorce.

Breastfeeding professionals know the important role a supportive father can play in the success of a breastfeeding relationship. Nursing mothers who experience marital separation and divorce during pregnancy or their children's infancy may suffer from the lack of direct spousal support and experience additional challenges to the maintenance of breastfeeding created by the added burden of custody arrangements and visitation schedules. Women who want to maintain their breastfeeding relationships through divorce often face inconsistent and unclear advice as to whether and/or how the legal system will consider breast-feeding as a factor in the allocation of parenting time (Sweet, 2010). Though there are some exceptions, family court systems in the United States are not adequately equipped with appropriate information to make consistent rulings that include maintenance of the breastfeeding relationship as a relevant factor in these decisions.

Child Custody and the Role of Parenting Plans

The term custody includes both legal custody, which is the ability of a parent to make decisions for the child, and physical custody, which refers to the physical possession of the child (Atkinson, 2000). In the United States, stability in the child's residential environment is prioritized, and rarely will even joint custody allocate a child's residential time to fifty-fifty with each parent (Schepard, 2004). Typically, even when parents share joint legal custody, one parent will retain primary physical custody of the child. The parent without primary physical custody will then have visitation rights to ensure an ongoing relationship with the child. Even though courts no longer presume the mother is the most fit residential parent, in practice, mothers retain primary physical custody in up to 90% of divorces (Silverstein, 1996), and for purposes of this paper, we will assume, as is typically the case, that the mother is the breastfeeding child's primary physical custodian.

Since the traditional language of custody and visitation tends to increase parental conflict by creating a winner and a loser in the post-divorce parenting scheme, many jurisdictions have switched to the concept of parenting plans, which attempt to encourage the emergence of cooperative co-parenting relationships, post-divorce (Schepard, 2004). As parents are better equipped than the court to evaluate their own unique parenting circumstances, parents will ideally negotiate parenting plans on their own, with the court stepping in only when they are unable to reach mutual agreement. Research has consistently shown that level of parent conflict is one of the largest factors relating to a child's adaptability and success, post-divorce (McKnight & Erickson, 2004), so recent family law trends have been in the direction of encouraging parental cooperation and reducing the conflict inherent in repeated and drawn out court battles over custody.

Many courts, bar organizations, and commentators have developed parenting plan information sheets, forms, and guidelines for use in their jurisdictions. Even though relatively few custody arrangements are actually litigated in court, these standard parenting plan documents are very important to the actual child custody determinations made both in and out of court. First of all, a very large number of the divorces handled today are handled *prose*, or without the parties hiring attorneys and standardized forms have the advantage of offering a framework for such applicants to develop appropriate plans (American Bar Association, 2001). Furthermore, parenting plan guidelines often provide a legal baseline that informs the parties' decision-making in alternative dispute resolution processes, such as mediation and collaborative law (Murphy & Rubinson, 2009). From a practical perspective, when a father knows the minimum visitation that would be ordered in a court ruling, the mother may have little actual ability to negotiate for less visitation in order to best accommodate breastfeeding schedules.

The goal of this paper is to detail the kinds of accommodations for breastfeeding that divorcing mothers can expect to see in typical parenting plan guidelines actually used in the U.S. legal system. Though breastfeeding has a valuable role in fostering mother-child attachment and bonding, and there are substantial reasons to support breastfeeding from the perspective of a child's emotional development (U.S. Department of Health and Human Services, 2011), this paper focuses on the nutritive aspects of breastfeeding for the simple reason that it is what the courts do (Hofheimer, 1998). This is not an attempt to propose model accommodations for breastfeeding in parenting plans, and many of the guidelines described in this paper reflect either severe information gaps with regards to breastfeeding or most typically, fail to consider it as a factor at all. Mothers with low-conflict relationships with their ex-spouses, or with ex-spouses who are supportive of breastfeeding, may be able to negotiate parenting plans that take the needs of their breastfeeding child into greater account.

Real parenting plans in any given jurisdiction may be more or less protective of breastfeeding than what is described below, depending on applicable statutes, case law, the biases of individual participants in the process, and the unique fact scenarios involved. Furthermore, parents with multiple children will face added issues of accommodating the age-based needs of different siblings.

Breastfeeding Infants Under 6 Months of Age

Generally, exclusively breastfed infants under 6 months of age are the most likely to have their breastfeeding status taken into account with regards to visitation or alternatively to have parenting plans that favor preservation of breastfeeding, even when breastfeeding is not an explicit factor.

Several parenting plan guidelines explicitly take breastfeeding into account. A parenting plan guide used in Massachusetts suggests that for children under 9 months of age, "parents should consider the special needs of breastfeeding infants" (Massachusetts Association of Family and Conciliation Courts). Likewise, a model plan used in Utah suggests that parents should consider the needs of breastfed infants in making parenting plans (Utah State Courts). Unfortunately, neither plan offers suggestions as to how breastfeeding should be factored into the decision-making process.

Even when breastfeeding status is not explicitly accounted for, most jurisdictions tend to structure parenting plans for infants under 6 months old in ways that are protective of breastfeeding. The common preference for "short frequent visits" with the non-residential parent for young infants rather than "longer visits spaced farther apart" (Indiana Supreme Court, 2008) is appropriate from the perspective of lactation physiology. The guidelines used by the Los Angeles Superior Court are typical of those including developmental considerations without regards to breastfeeding, recommending for all infants visits of "three non-consecutive days per week for two hours each day" for the ages of birth to 6 months (Los Angeles Superior Court, 2007). Regular visits of 2 to 3 hours each offer the father and infant the benefit of regular contact, but are short enough to minimally impact the breastfeeding relationship. Many breastfeeding mothers will be able to accommodate such visits without even having to resort to expressing milk, though most guidelines do suggest shared caregiving responsibility, including feeding, as a goal (Massachusetts Association of Family and Conciliation Courts).

Some guidelines mention breastfeeding, but do not suggest it as a factor to be accounted for in plans. Arizona's parenting plan guide mentions breastfeeding, but largely as a caution to mothers not to use breastfeeding as a reason to preclude paternal access:

> Parents who are not raising their child together must balance the baby's need to nurse with its need to bond with the father. The parents should talk often and openly with each other about the baby. Breastfeeding shouldn't be used to stop the father from spending time with the child. Instead, mothers need to offer the father parenting time, and fathers need to be flexible regarding the need of the baby to nurse. The father can feed an infant with the mother's expressed (pumped) milk, particularly after nursing routines are well established (Arizona Supreme Court, 2009).

Similarly, a guide to developmentally appropriate parenting plans published by the ABA suggests that from 0 to 4 months, "if breastfeeding is chosen as the primary method of feeding at birth (unless committed to strict La Leche League standards), a bottle or nipple substitute could be introduced within the first month or two" (Hartson & Payne, 2006). While not particularly attuned to the maintenance of at-the-breast-feeding, as opposed to breast-milk feeding, this guide recommends visitation with the non-residential parent of 2 to 3 hours several days a week, with no extended or overnight visits, a schedule that does serve to allow a father frequent interaction with his child, with minimal interruption to breastfeeding. As these guides demonstrate, parenting plans tend to focus on the nutritional aspects of breastfeeding (Sweet & Power, 2009), and fail to consider the psychosocial effects, which may be the most important factors in a woman's decision to breastfeed (U.S. Department of Health and Human Services, 2011).

Breastfeeding Infants between 6 to 12 Months of Age

Sometime in the 6-to-12-months-age range, many jurisdictions will start adding overnight visitation with the nonresidential parent to the parenting time allocation. Overnight visitations present a unique challenge in the context of breastfeeding, as the length of mother-baby separation will require the mother to express her milk, or run the risk of discomfort, pain, and supply reduction. Some mothers will be able to accommodate this additional pumping with relative ease, but for many, overnight separations signal the beginning of the end of the nursing relationship (Sweet & Power, 2009).

Overnight visitation for young children has been one of the most hotly debated issues in family law in recent years. As it has evolved in recent years, attachment theory now emphasizes the possibility of multiple early attachments, rather than attachment to only one primary caregiver, and there is a substantial body of psychological research documenting the benefits to the child that result from increased paternal involvement in caregiving roles, post-divorce. As summarized by Warshak (2000):

> Contemporary attachment theory has abandoned the notion of "monotropy"—the idea that children have a

biological need to develop a selective attachment with just one person. The notion that children have only one psychological parent has been thoroughly discredited by a large body of evidence which has demonstrated that infants normally develop close attachments to both of their parents, that this occurs at about the same time (approximately 6 months of age), and that they do best when they have the opportunity to establish and maintain such attachments.

There has been quite a bit of debate in academic circles about the implications the changes in attachment theory have for overnight visitation, with some commentators still favoring blanket restrictions on overnight visits for young children (Solomon & Biringen, 2001), while many now argue that infants thrive with early overnight visitation (Kelly & Lamb, 2000; Pruett et al., 2004).

This growing body of research, combined with changes in women's roles in our society in recent decades, has resulted in an explicit rejection of the old "tender years doctrine," which presumed young children were best off with their mothers after divorce (Schepard, 2004). Modern courts are typically hostile to arguments against overnight visitation that are rooted in the notion of the primacy of the mother-baby relationship. Thus, in the current climate, any argument limiting overnight visitation for breastfed babies is best articulated for reasons other than the mother-baby attachment.

Unless a non-custodial parent has been uninvolved in a child's care before the separation, most parenting plan guidelines begin to add overnight visitation as an option at some point before the child's first birthday. Los Angeles guidelines suggest expanding visitation in the 7 to 12 months age range to "three non-consecutive days per week for three hours each day" and "overnight, if appropriate," with no discussion of breastfeeding as a factor limiting the appropriateness of overnight visits (Los Angeles Superior Court, 2007). Indiana's parenting time guidelines suggest that unless a non-custodial parent has not had regular care for the child, "parenting time shall include overnight," and includes the possibility of overnight visits starting at birth (Indiana Supreme Court, 2008).

Even those guidelines that explicitly protect breast-feeding for the young infant get noticeably less protective as the infant ages. The Massachusetts guidelines mentioned above, for example, only apply to infants under 9 months of age. In its discussion of the needs of breastfeeding infants between ages of 4 and 8 months, the American Bar Association publication on creating developmentally appropriate parenting plans moves away from special accommodations for breastfeeding, asserting that "even if an infant was breastfed exclusively prior to 4 months, most mothers express breastmilk by this time in order to return to work or mix with cereal (most infants start cereal in addition to formula or breastmilk at about 4 months)" (Hartson & Payne, 2006), advice contrary to the recommended 6 months of exclusive breastfeeding before the introduction of solid foods promulgated by the American Academy of Pediatrics and World Health Organization. Hartson and Payne's developmental guidelines begin overnight visits in the 4 to 8 months age range, and stop mentioning breastfeeding as a factor after 8 months.

Breastfeeding Infants/Toddlers Over 12 Months of Age

Breastfed infants over 12 months of age are the least likely to have their breastfeeding status taken into account in custody determinations. Breastfeeding past 1 year of age is the exception, rather than the norm in the United States (U.S. Department of Health and Human Services, 2011). Despite the plentiful evidence of health and emotional benefits to nursing beyond 1 year, courts are much less likely to consider breastfeeding truly necessary for infants over 1 year of age, especially if it conflicts with paternal access to the child.

While the author has not been able to find any parenting plan breastfeeding protections explicitly applying to children over 12 months, some guidelines do include breastfeeding as a factor without age limitations. A proposed parenting plan used by one Hawaii court lists "breastfeeding infant," without regard to age, as a special concern to consider in drafting parenting plans (State of Hawaii Family Court: First Circuit, 2005). Michigan's Parenting Time Guideline has perhaps the most expansive protection of breastfeeding of any jurisdiction in its discussion of special factors for children under school age:

By statute, the age of child(ren) is a factor when the child(ren) is receiving substantial nutrition through nursing. If the child(ren) is nursing, the parenting time shall be limited and arranged in a manner to accommodate the nursing pattern unless other provisions can be made (Michigan State Court Administrative Office).

Though Michigan's statute does include an age limit of 12 months for considering breastfeeding as a factor (Mich. coMp. Laws § 722.27a (2009)), the parenting time guidelines notably do not, though this may simply be due to oversight of the possibility that a child over 12 months could still be "receiving substantial nutrition through nursing."

Even with regular overnight separations, some mothers of toddlers are able to find ways to sustain their nursing relationships in spite of separations. If a mother is able to express her milk through separations, and her child is willing to nurse when he is with his mother and not nurse when he they are apart, a mother may find this kind of extended nursing strategy particularly empowering of her continued unique role in her child's life, post-divorce (Sweet, 2010). Lactation consultants can be of particular help in this context, assisting mothers in developing strategies to sustain breastfeeding through regular overnight separations.

References

American Bar Association: Center for Professional Responsibility (2010). *Model rules of professional conduct R. 1.2.* Washington, DC: American Bar Association. Retrieved from http://goo.gl/VG57YB

American Bar Association: Center on Children and the Law (2001). *A judge's guide: Making child-centered custody decisions in custody cases.* Chicago, IL: American Bar Association.

Arizona Supreme Court, Court Services Division, Court Programs Unit. (2009). *Planning for parenting time: Arizona's guide for parents living apart.* Retrieved from http://azcourts.gov/Portals/31/ParentingTime/ PPWguidelines.pdf

Atkinson, J. (2000). *Modern child custody practice (2nd Ed.)* New Providence, N.J.: Matthew Bender & Company.

Hartson, J., & Payne, B. (2006) *Creating effective parenting plans: A developmental approach for lawyers and divorce professionals.* Chicago, IL: American Bar Association Section of Family Law.

Hofheimer, K. D. (1998). Breastfeeding as a factor in child custody and visitation decisions. *Virginia Journal of Social Policy and Law, 5,* 433.

Indiana Supreme Court. (2008). *Indiana rules of court: Indiana parenting time guidelines.* Retrieved from http://www.in.gov/judiciary/rules/parenting/ index.html

Kelly, J.B., & Lamb, M.E. (2000). Using child development research to make appropriate custody and access decisions for young children. *Family & Conciliation Courts Review, 38,* 297-331.

Los Angeles Superior Court. (2007). *Creating a parenting plan: Children under three.* Retrieved from http://www.lasuperiorcourt.org/familylaw/pdfs/ parentingunder3.pdf

Massachussetts Association of Family and Conciliation Courts. *Planning for shared parenting: A guide for parents living apart.* Retrieved from http:// www.mass.gov/courts/courtsandjudges/courts/probateandfamilycourt/ afccsharedparenting.pdf

McKnight, M. S., & Erickson, S. K. (2004). The plan to separately parent children after divorce. In J. Folberg, A. L. Milne, & P. Salem (Eds.), *Divorce and family mediation: Models, techniques and applications* (pp. 129-154). New York: The Guilford Press.

Me. *Rev. Stat. tit.* 19, § 1653(3)(P). (2011). Available at http://www. mainelegislature.org/legis/statutes/19-A/title19-Asec1653.html

Mich. Comp. Laws § 722.27a. (2009). Available at http://www. legislature. mi.gov/(S(zly4ak55ma2prjjhkfayox55))/mileg. aspx?page=getobject&objec tname=mcl-722-27a

Michigan State Court Administrative Office. *Michigan parenting time guideline.* Retrieved from http://www.courts.michigan.gov/ scao/resources/ publications/manuals/focb/pt_gdlns.pdf

Murphy, J., & Rubinson, R. (2009). *Family mediation: Theory and practice.* New Providence, N.J.: Matthew Bender & Company.

National Conference of State Legislatures. *Breastfeeding laws* (updated May 2011). Available at http://www.ncsl.org/default. aspx?tabid=14389

Pruett, M. K., Arthur, L.A., & Ebling, R. (2007). The hand that rocks the cradle: Maternal gatekeeping after divorce. *Pace Law Review, 27,* 704-739.

Pruett, M.K., Ebling, R., & Insabella, G. (2004). Critical aspects of parenting plans for young children: Interjecting data into the debate about overnight. *Family Court Review, 42,* 39-59.

Schepard, A. I. (2004). Children, courts and custody: *Interdisciplinary models for divorcing families.* Cambridge, UK: Cambridge University Press.

Seltzer, J. A., Schaeffer, N. C., & Charng, H. (1989). Family ties after divorce: The relationship between visiting and paying child support. *Journal of Marriage and Family, 51,* 1013-1031.

Silverstein, L.B. (1996). Fathering is a feminist issue. *Psychology of Women Quarterly, 20,* 3-37.

Solomon, J., & Biringen, Z. (2001). Another look at the developmental research: Commentary on Kelly and Lamb's "Using child development research to make appropriate custody and access decisions for young children." *Family Court Review, 39,* 355-364.

State of Hawaii Family Court: First Circuit. (2005). *Proposed parenting plan.* Retrieved from http://www.courts.state.hi.us/ docs/docs1/ propparentplan030206mod.pdf

Sweet, L. (2010). Breastfeeding throughout legal separation: Women's experiences of the Australian Family Law System. *Journal of Human Lactation, 26*, 384-392.

Sweet, L., & Power, C. (2009). Family Law as a determinant of child health and welfare: Shared parenting, breastfeeding, and the best interests of the child. *Health Sociology Review, 18*, 108-118.

U.S. Department of Health and Human Services, U.S. Public Health Service, Office of the Surgeon General (2011). *The Surgeon General's Call to Action to Support Breastfeeding.* Retrieved from http://www.surgeongeneral.gov/ topics/breastfeeding/ calltoactiontosupportbreastfeeding.pdf

Utah Code $ 30-3-34(2)(n). (2008). Available at http://le.utah. gov/~code/ TITLE30/htm/30_03_003400.htm

Utah State Courts. *Pointers for parents and parenting plans.* Retrieved from http://utcourts.gov/howto/family/parenting_plans/docs/99_Pointers_for_Parents_and_Parenting_Plans.pdf

Warshak, R.A. (2000). Blanket restrictions: Overnight contact between parents and young children. *Family and Conciliation Courts Review, 38*, 422-445.

Late Preterm Infant Toolkit

The Oklahoma Infant Alliance has created these guidelines for health care providers and families, promoting better understanding of the issues concerning these just-a-little-too-early infants, born between 34 and 37 weeks gestation. The toolkit addresses both medical issues, as well as emotional issues that impact the families. To see sample pages from the toolkit and to order a copy, go to http://oklahomainfantalliance.org/lpi_guidelines.html.

Toward Improving the Outcome of Pregnancy III

Toward Improving the Outcome of Pregnancy: Enhancing Perinatal Health Through Quality, Safety and Performance Initiatives is a free report available from the March of Dimes. It explores the elements that are essential to improving quality, safety and performance across the continuum of perinatal care: consistent data collection and measurement; evidence-based initiatives; adherence to clinical practice guidelines; a life-course perspective; care that is patient- and family-centered, culturally sensitive, and linguistically appropriate; policies that support high-quality perinatal care; and systems change.

Ultimately, reaching a more efficient, more accountable system of perinatal care will require a level of collaboration, services integration and communication that lead to successful perinatal quality improvement initiatives, many which are described throughout this book. In addition to the consistent collection of data and measurement and the application of evidence-based interventions, successful collaborations, like all perinatal quality improvement, depend on the engagement, support and commitment of everyone reading this book: health care professionals and hospital leadership, public-health professionals, and community-based service providers, research scientists, policy-makers and payers, as well as patients and families.

http://www.marchofdimes.com/professionals/medicalresources_tiop.html

USLCA

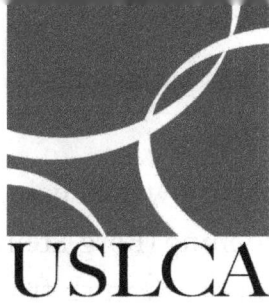

Preventing Musculoskeletal Pain in Mothers

Ergonomic Tips for Lactation Consultants

Debbie Roberts, MA, OTR/L[1]

Keywords: postpartum, nerve entrapment, ergonomics, musculoskeletal disorders, positioning, posture, pain

Physiologic and postural changes that occur during pregnancy and the postpartum period, combined with the physical demands of infant care, may place women at risk for musculoskeletal pain and musculoskeletal disorders (MSDs). Lactation consultants, working in conjunction with occupational and physical therapists, are in a unique position to teach postpartum women how to incorporate ergonomic principles into breastfeeding and daily infant care.

Pregnancy and the postpartum period are associated with physiologic changes that can predispose a woman toward developing musculoskeletal pain. Physiologic changes in pregnancy include soft-tissue edema, increased fluid

1   johnroberts@pol.net

retention, ligament laxity, weight gain, hyperlordosis, and symphysis pubis widening (Borg-Stein et al., 2005, p. 182). These physiologic changes can shift a woman's center of gravity, resulting in both overstretching and shortening of postural muscles. For example, "anterior shoulder muscles, lumbar paraspinals and hip flexors" typically shorten while abdominal and pelvic floor muscles tend to overstretch or weaken (Hall & Brody, 2005, p. 266). Tight neck and shoulder muscles combined with overstretched abdominals and paraspinal muscles may predispose a postpartum woman toward adopting a kyphotic posture when breastfeeding. Kyphotic positioning (head forward, shoulders protracted) can cause "significant intradiskal pressure increases and potential mictrotrauma to spinal tissues" (Speicher et al., 2006).

Up until 12 weeks postpartum, a woman may continue to be at risk for joint hypermobility due to the influence of hormones on ligaments and connective tissue (Hall & Brody, 2005, p. 266). During pregnancy:

> [It] is estimated that virtually all women experience some degree of musculoskeletal discomfort ... and 25% have at least temporarily disabling symptoms. Lower back pain is the most common impairment, affecting 50% of pregnant women. Other common disorders include pelvic pain, upper- and lower-extremity pain, and peripheral neuropathy (Borg-Stein & Dugan, 2007, p. 459).

Women may also develop pain in the postpartum period due to the "continued hormonal influence of lactation on the musculoskeletal system [combined] with the biomechanical and ergonomic stresses of childcare-related activities" (Borg Stein & Dugan, 2007, p. 472). This article will review some of the common pain syndromes experienced by postpartum women, discuss ergonomic considerations as applied to breastfeeding education, and provide positioning suggestions that may help prevent postpartum musculoskeletal pain.

Musculoskeletal pain in the postpartum period may be influenced by pre-existing medical conditions, and by the sleep deprivation associated with infant care. Pre-existing conditions, such as depression, degenerative joint disease, chronic pain syndromes, and immune system disorders, may increase postpartum muscle and joint discomfort. For example, hypothyroidism may predispose a postpartum mother toward developing carpal tunnel or tarsal tunnel syndrome (Ashworth, 2008; Peira & Brown, 2008). Sleep deprivation augments acute pain, decreases pressure pain tolerance (muscle and skin nociception), increases sensitivity to noxious stimuli, increases fatigue and negative mood, and decreases cognition (Lautenbacher et al., 2006).

The terms musculoskeletal disorder (MSD), musculoskeletal pain, cumulative trauma disorder (CTD), over-use syndromes, repetitive strain injuries, cervicobrachial disorders, and repetitive motion injuries are considered descriptive, not diagnostic. Some CTDs, such as DeQuervain's syndrome, have a clear diagnosis and can be linked to specific physical stressors (Mackin et al., 2002). In the setting of postpartum care, women should be referred to their primary care provider to confirm or rule out any underlying medical conditions. If appropriate, her primary care provider may order additional evaluations or therapy services.

Postpartum recommendations for daily physical activities, such as lifting, are also under scrutiny and may be too restrictive (Minig et al., 2009). In the absence of well-defined activity limitations, allied health professionals may need to place a greater emphasis on prevention and early referral for additional services when a postpartum mother presents with musculoskeletal pain. Lactation consultants are in a unique position to model ergonomic principles during breastfeeding and daily infant-care activities. Practitioners may also experience the benefits firsthand, since ergonomic goals focus on joint protection, proper body mechanics, energy conservation, and activity modification.

In this setting, an ergonomic assessment conducted by an occupational or physical therapist includes a chart review and interview to determine risk factors, a sensory-motor evaluation, if indicated, and an observation of the breastfeeding session. An occupational therapist would observe the mother, baby, lactation consultant, and the set-up (i.e., furniture, equipment, and tools of the trade). General recommendations focus on finding the optimal position for the mother, baby, and lactation consultant. Optimal positioning for an adult can be envisioned as a neutral position that promotes balanced posture and avoids musculoskeletal strain. A neutral spine position refers to "the most comfortable spinal position for the individual to complete movement patterns and then integrate this neutral position in daily occupations. The neutral position for each individual is the condition under which the vertebrae and discs are under equal pressure" (Pendleton & Schultz-Krohn, 2006, p. 1040).

A neutral forearm position can be envisioned when an individual stands with arms hanging, relaxed, by the side, with palms facing towards the individual's thighs and thumbs facing forward. When the individual sits or flexes the elbows, the thumbs now point towards the ceiling. Achieving a neutral forearm position depends heavily on the individual's general posture. For example, slumping forward may internally rotate the shoulder and pronate the forearm. Thus, it's more effective to position the trunk first, in order to provide a stable base of support for distal movements in the arm. Optimal positioning for the infant focuses on physiologic flexion. This is the stable base of support that promotes feeding. Envision sucking, swallowing, and breathing as the distal movement.[2]

---

2   This concept is a basic tenet of Neuro-Developmental Treatment or NDT. "Proper alignment of body segments is important for postural control. Alignment is a core element of movement that requires a base of support, a healthy soft-tissue system, structural integrity of the joints, and adequate range of motion. Ideal alignment results in optimal length-tension relationships for muscle fibers, increasing the potential for muscle activation" (Pendleton & Schultlz-Krohn, 2006, p. 771).

General Principles of Energy Conservation

» Simplify tasks.

» Organize work spaces to eliminate unnecessary bending, twisting, lifting, and carrying.

» Roll or slide objects rather than carrying or lifting them.

» Pace the day with frequent rest breaks. Rest while the baby sleeps. Rest after eating. Rest before becoming overly fatigued.

» Sit instead of stand, as sitting requires less energy expenditure than standing.

» Use gravity-eliminated positions that require less energy expenditure.

Putting it into Practice

A side-lying position with a pillow placed between her knees or ankles is a gravity-eliminated position that promotes a neutral spine position and minimizes fatigue during breastfeeding (Milligan et al., 1996). Resting or breastfeeding in this position may help the mother conserve energy. If the mother has pre-existing spinal disease, generalized weakness, or muscle tone deviations (hyper- or hypotonia), side-lying may be a preferred position to breastfeed. Place a pillow between her knees and ankles to promote neutral spinal alignment. Additional pillows may be used to support her upper body in neutral alignment and to provide back support.

General Principles of Joint Protection and Proper Body Mechanics

» Avoid using a sustained, tight grasp or pinch, especially if the wrist is bent.

» Avoid static or awkward positions for prolonged periods.

» Minimize repetition.

» Avoid bending, extending, or twisting the wrist during activities.

» Use a power grasp (loose grip, keeping all the fingers together, thumb straight).

» Avoid reaching, grasping, and lifting with the palm down (especially with wrist bent). Rather, support objects from underneath with the palm up (wrist straight).

» Avoid leaning over a work surface or twisting the torso while lifting.

When lifting and carrying, keep objects close to the body. Keep a straight back. Use a wide base of support (feet spread apart). Use leg muscles to lift from a squatting, kneeling, or half-kneeling position (may not be appropriate for all postpartum women). Use a golfer's lift; bend at the hips while raising one leg behind (Pendleton & Schultz-Krohn, 2006).

Putting it into Practice

Carrying the Baby

When lifting a baby, scoop one hand under the baby's bottom, and use your other forearm to support the body. Avoid lifting the baby from under the armpits. This increases the risk of thumb tendonitis by placing the wrist in ulnar deviation and the thumb into extension. If the baby is on the floor, kneel, and bring your baby close to your chest before standing.

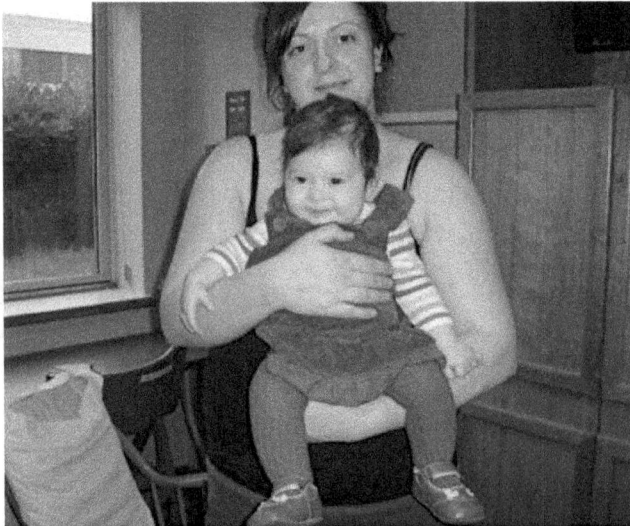

Figure 1. Carrying a heavy baby.

When carrying a heavy baby, keep one hand and forearm under the baby's bottom, and use the other arm to support the baby's trunk. This also keeps the baby's shoulders protracted and allows the baby to use both hands in midline (See Figure 1).

Avoid carrying the baby on one hip. This places stress on the mother's pelvis and promotes shoulder retraction in the baby. Instead, consider using a sling with padded shoulder supports or a baby-pack to support the baby's weight.

Avoid carrying the baby in a portable car seat! Especially avoid using only one hand to carry the car seat. Instead, push the baby in a stroller or carry the baby manually (American College of Sports Medicine, 2006; Hajic, 2010). If you must carry the car seat, use two hands and keep it close to your chest. If using a stroller, consider adjusting the height of the handles to keep the individual's wrist straight. If the stroller seat reclines, the baby may enjoy a position change. Sitting in a car seat flexes infant hip muscles, while a reclined or semi-reclined position allows the infant to stretch hip-flexor muscles.

Carrying an infant manually may also promote symmetrical head-shaping and strengthen the infant's neck and shoulder musculature (Hummel & Fortado, 2005). For example, positioning the baby with his or her forearms resting against the mother's chest provides a modified tummy-time position for the baby, and allows the mother to support the baby's bottom with one forearm and support the baby's back with her other arm. Both the mother and baby have a symmetrical posture and the baby gets a little upper body, head, and neck strengthening. The American Occupational Therapy Association, the American Physical Therapy Association, and the American Academy of Pediatrics highly recommend giving infants a variety of positioning experiences in order to get enough supervised tummy-time throughout the day (Block, 2008; Pathways Awareness Foundation Brochure, 2011; Pin et al., 2007; Waitzman, 2007).

Bottle-feeding

When bottle-feeding, consider that placing the baby in side-lying position may have biomechanical advantages for both the baby and the person feeding the infant. Side-lying is a gravity-eliminated plane that may provide the safest position to bottle-feed expressed breast milk to a baby who has feeding or swallowing difficulties (Obvious exceptions include a baby who presents cleft lip or palate). Placing the baby in side-lying position can also help the feeder pace the "flow" of EBM from the bottle, which may help protect future breastfeedings (Goldfield et al., 2006; Shaker, 2010; Wolf & Glass, 2011).

First, seat the mother in a slightly reclined position. For a righthanded mother, place a pillow under her left forearm so that it touches the back of the chair, yet extends past her fingertips. Her left forearm and shoulder should feel supported. Next, position the baby on his or her left side so that the baby's back rests against the mother's left forearm and the baby's neck and shoulders are supported by the mother's hand. The baby's feet may touch the back of the chair or mother's arm, depending on his or her size. The mother's hand should be relaxed and open, and the wrist straight. The mother should avoid supporting the baby's head in the web-space of her hand. The mother should be able to relax her shoulders back into the chair. This position discourages the mother from slumping her back and dropping her head forward, which could lead to neck, and upper and mid-back pain (Jeffcoat, 2009). This position simultaneously protects the joints and ligaments in the left arm. The mother should avoid holding the bottle with a tight grip and wrist flexion with her right hand.

When selecting a bottle, consider its shape, weight, and the size of the mother's hand. In general, avoid a wide, heavy bottle. If the infant requires a cleft-palate bottle system, consider how much effort the feeder needs to exert in order to control flow rate. For example, the Mead Johnson Cleft Palate Nurser is ovoid in shape (which may challenge small hands), and is made of flexible plastic. In order to control flow rate and assist with swallowing, the feeder's hand squeezes the bottle in relation to the baby's sucking/breathing rhythm (Wiet et al., 2010). This repetitive, squeezing motion may place stress on hand tendons and joints. In contrast, the Haberman Feeder (Medela) may offer an ergonomic advantage. It has a thinner, cylindrical shape, a one-way valve system that reduces air intake, and a specially designed nipple that allows for three flow rates. If the baby needs help extracting liquid, the feeder can gently squeeze the nipple.

Selecting Clothing

When selecting clothing, keep it simple for both the mother and baby. Choose infant clothing that has few buttons or snaps. For example, an infant gown with drawstring closure may simplify nighttime diaper changes. A two-piece outfit may be easier to manipulate than a one-piece outfit that has multiple snaps (Hajic, 2010). Velcro fasteners may be easier to manipulate than snaps, safety pins, or buttons. The mother should also choose simple outfits for herself to minimize buttoning, snapping, and the need to re-arrange clothing in preparation for nursing. Specialty clothing that facilitates Kangaroo-Care holding, or nursing bras that fasten in the front, may be helpful. Choosing the right nursing bra– supportive but not tight—is equally important. An ill-fitting bra may produce pain, tingling, or numbness in the cervical spine, thoracic spine, shoulder, arm, or hand.

Mothers' Position While Sitting

When breastfeeding, discourage the mother from crossing her legs or placing one ankle across the opposite knee,

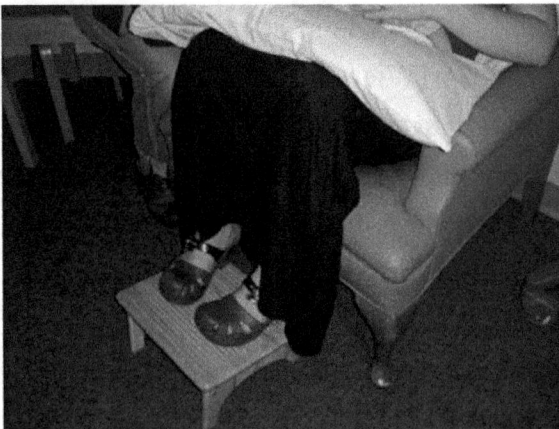

Figure 2.

Semi-reclined, seated position with knees slightly higher than hips.

since this stresses the ligaments in her lower back, pelvis, and knee. If seated in a chair, use a footstool to position the mother's flexed knees slightly higher than her hips. This promotes a semi-reclined position (See Figure 2).

If the mother is semi-reclined in bed or in a reclining chair, she may need a small pillow or rolled towel placed against her low back to achieve a comfortable, neutral spine position. There are several benefits to this position. A semi-reclined position uses gravity to help hold the baby in position, which decreases the amount of force that the mother needs to exert in order to support the baby. The mother's nipple will be in a more upright position, which should decrease the amount of hand force she needs to exert in order to support her breast. This semi-reclined breastfeeding position may also help the baby achieve a self-latch (Colson et al., 2008) (See Figure 3).

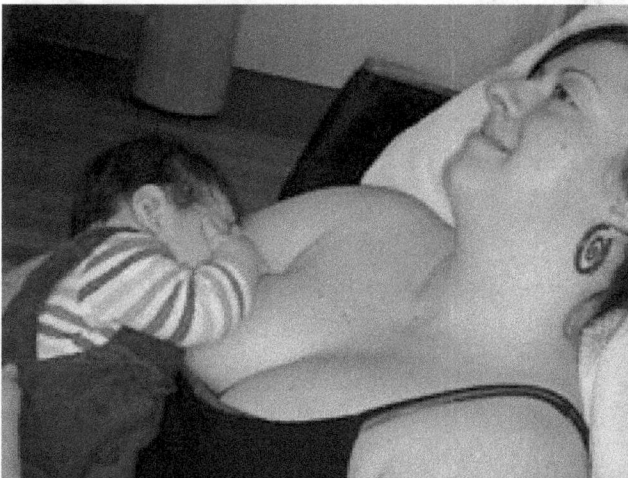

Figure 3. Semi-reclined breastfeeding position with the mother's shoulders and forearms in a relaxed posture.

Discourage the mother from leaning forward to bring the breast to the baby since this produces shoulder protraction and could lead to "increased strain on the posterior neck and upper back muscles while the muscles in the front of the neck and shoulders are placed in a shortened position, causing them to lose flexibility over time" (Jeffcoat, 2009, p. 30). Rather, encourage the mother to bring the baby up to her breast as described in the section describing a semi-reclined breastfeeding position. Look for symmetry, and remember that a neutral position should be relaxing and comfortable (See Figure 4).

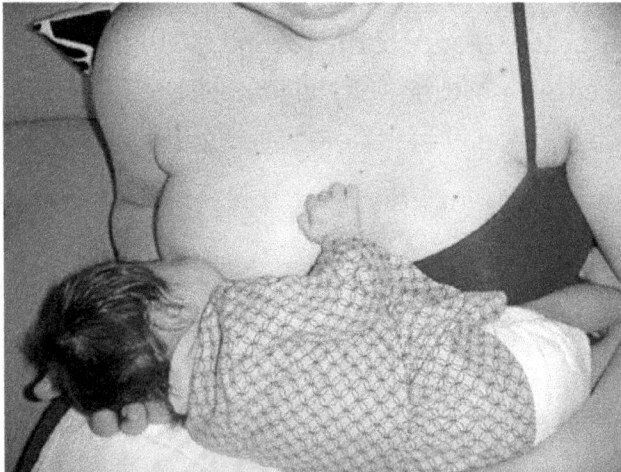

Figure 4. The mother is leaning forward, producing a slumped-shoulder position that may lead to neck, upper-back, and midback pain. The baby's head is acting as a compressive force on the mother's hand, which may lead to hand, wrist, forearm, or shoulder pain.

Placing a flat pillow under the infant and under the mother's forearm or wrist may help promote a neutral wrist and forearm position when using a cross-cradle hold or football hold. A premature infant, small-for-gestational-age infant, or infant with atypical muscle tone may also benefit from the extra support of a breastfeeding pillow. If the mother has preexisting cervical, thoracic, or lumbar joint disease, she may need a rolled towel at the corresponding spinal level to achieve neutral, pain-free alignment. If she has nerve compression in the cervical spine or forearm, she may need additional pillow support for her forearm and shoulder (See Figure 5).

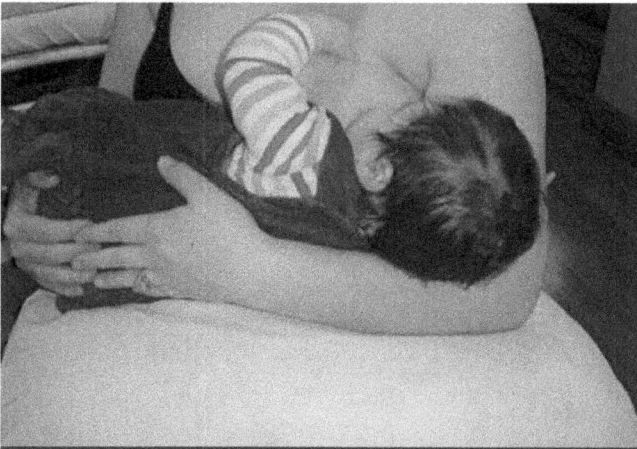

Figure 5. A flat pillow is providing support for the mother's forearm and shoulder. The mother's wrist, hand, and forearm appear to be in a relaxed and neutral position. The baby is also in a relaxed, neutral alignment that promotes age-appropriate flexion.

When performing breast compressions or when supporting the breast, encourage mothers to use the "C" hold rather than the "scissors hold" (See Figure 6). The "scissors hold" places more stress on the wrist extensor tendons (and potentially flexor tendons) since the mother's wrist is flexed, and her fingers must forcefully abduct against the breast tissue. This places the wrist and fingers at a biomechanical disadvantage— the wrist is in an awkward position while the fingers perform a repetitive, forceful pinch and grasp. Avoid long periods of time in which the mother supports her breast with one hand. Especially avoid resting the baby's head in the web-space of the mother's hand while the wrist is flexed. This compressive force may lead to Stenosing Tenosynovitis.

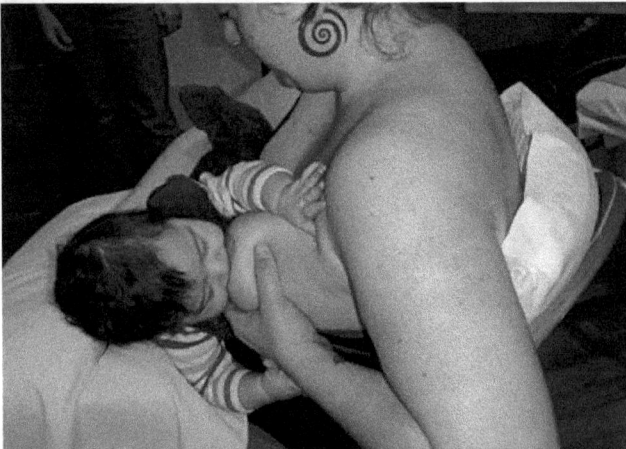

Figure 6. The mother using a "C" hold to simulate a breast compression. Note that her left wrist is in a neutral position. The baby is positioned symmetrically, with midline orientation of her hands.

General Positioning Tips

Don't worry about fixing every aspect of positioning, especially if the mother is comfortable and the baby is nursing well (See Figure 7).

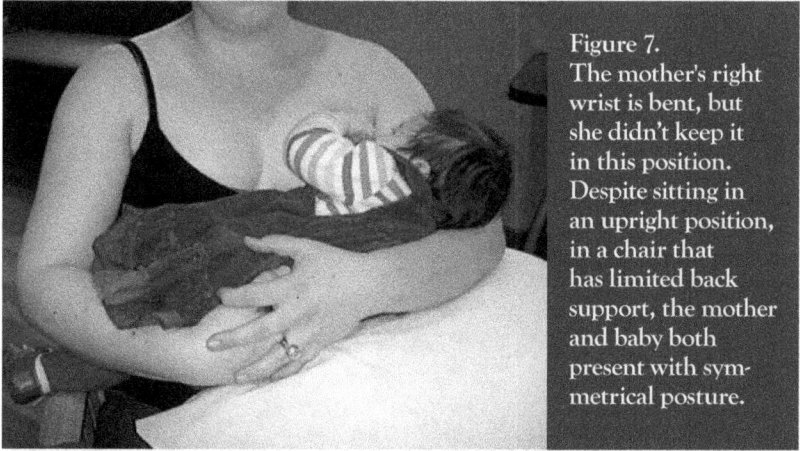

Figure 7. The mother's right wrist is bent, but she didn't keep it in this position. Despite sitting in an upright position, in a chair that has limited back support, the mother and baby both present with symmetrical posture.

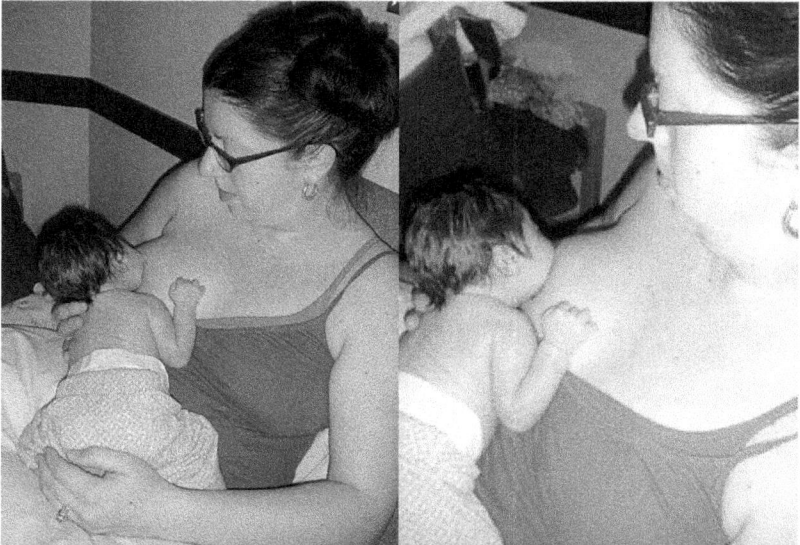

Figures 8 & 9. The mother's left hand and forearm are in a relaxed, neutral position. As the baby crawls higher onto the breast, the mother has less stress on her right hand and wrist.

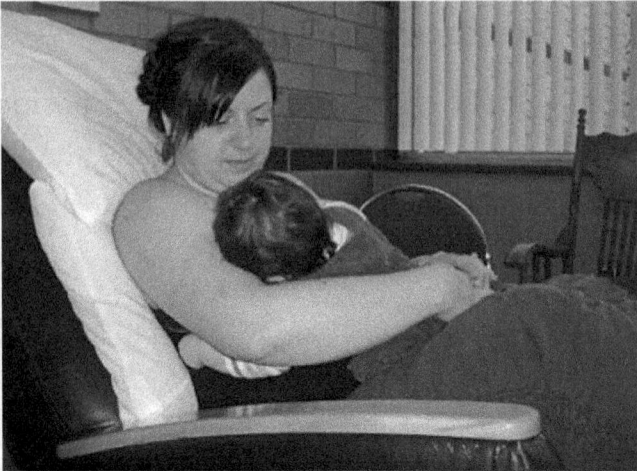

Figure 10. Sometimes the "right" pillow(s) make all of the difference. A softer, squishier pillow would have filled in the gap behind the mother's head and neck better than this thin pillow. A soft, squishy pillow placed under the mother's right arm would provide more support to her shoulder.

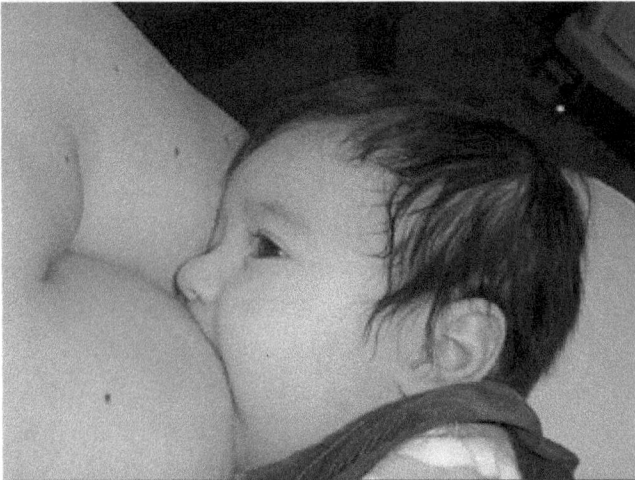

Figure 11. Once the mother understands the basic principles of positioning, she can problem solve on her own, freeing her to relax and enjoy her baby.

Conclusions

Lactation consultants, working in conjunction with occupational and physical therapists, can play an important role in teaching postpartum women how to incorporate proper body mechanics, joint protection, and energy conservation principles into breastfeeding and daily infant-care routines. New mothers who present with physical challenges, acute pain syndromes, or who present with unique infant feeding challenges, may also benefit from additional therapy services. Helping a new mother avoid awkward positioning that may lead to a musculo-skeletal pain disorder frees her to enjoy the everyday, quiet needs of her baby.

Special thanks to Maggie and Molly for modeling and to the lactation consultants at Evergreen Hospital, especially Jeanne Tate and Marie Witherall.

References

Ablove, R.H., & Ablove, T.S. (2009). Prevalence of carpal tunnel syndrome in pregnant women. *Women's Medical Journal, 108*(4), 194-196.

American College of Sports Medicine (ACSM). (2006). *Lifting while holding infant in carrier may result in lower back pain.* Press release from 53rd annual meeting. www.acsm.org/AM/Template. cfm?Section+Home Page&template=/CM/ContentDis...

Anderson, S.E., Steinbach, L.S., De Monaco, D., Bonel, H.M., Hurtienne, Y., & Voegelin, E. (2004). "Baby wrist": MRI of an overuse syndrome in mothers. *American Journal of Roentgenology, 182,* 719–724.

Ashworth, N.L. (2008). *Carpal tunnel syndrome.* Retrieved from http://www.emedicine.medscape.com.

Block, S. (2008). *Lack of time on tummy shown to hinder achievement of developmental milestones, say physical therapists.* News release, American Physical Therapy Association. Retrieved from http//: www.apta.org.

Borg-Stein, J., Dugan, S.A., & Gruber, J. (2005). Musculoskeletal aspects of pregnancy. *American Journal of Physical Medicine and Rehabilitation, 84*(3), 180-192.

Borg-Stein, J., & Dugan, S.A. (2007). Musculoskeletal disorders of pregnancy, delivery and postpartum. *Physical Medicine and Rehabilitation Clinics of North America, 18*(3), 459-476, ix.

Colson, S.D., Meek, J.H., & Hawdon, J.M. (2008). Optimal positions for the release of primitive neonatal reflexes stimulating breastfeeding. *Early Human Development, 84,* 441-449.

Goldfield, E.C., Richardson, M.J., Lee, K.G., & Margetts, S. (2006). Coordination of sucking, swallowing, and breathing, and oxygen saturation during early infant breastfeeding and bottle-feeding. *Pediatric Research, 60*(4), 450-455.

Hajic, M. (2010). *New parents at risk for RSI Pain.* BellaOnline The voice of women (Hixson, Ed). Retrieved from http://www. bellaonline.com.

Hall, C.M., & Brody, L.T. (2005). *Therapeutic exercise moving toward function, 2nd ed.* Philadelphia: Lippincott, Williams, & Wilkins.

Hummel, P., & Fortado, D. (2005). Impacting infant head shapes. *Advances in Neonatal Care, 5*(6), 329-340. Retrieved from http:// www.medscape.com

Jeffcoat, H. (2009). Help for postural pain after breastfeeding. *International Journal of Childbirth Education, 24*(1), 30-31.

Lautenbacher, S.L., Kundermann, B., & Krieg, J.C. (2006). Sleep deprivation and pain perception. *Sleep Medicine Reviews,* 10, 357-369.

Mackin E.J., Callahan, A.D., Skirven, T.M., Schneider, L.H., Osterman, A.L., & Hunter J.M. (Eds). (2002). *Rehabilitation of the hand and upper extremity, 5th ed.,* Vol. 1. St. Louis, MO: Mosby.

Milligan, R.A., Flenniken, P.M., & Pugh, L.C. (1996). Positioning intervention to minimize fatigue in breastfeeding women. *Applied Nursing Research, 9*(2), 67-70.

Minig, L., Trimble, E.L., Sarsotti, C., Sebastiani, M.M., & Spong, C.Y. (2009). Building the evidence base for postoperative and postpartum advice. *Obstetrics and Gynecology*, 114(4), 892-900.

Motion terminology images. Retrieved and reprinted with permission from http://www.ASSH.org. Also available in book form: Burton, Richard (chairman), 1983. *The hand: Examination and diagnosis*, 2*nd ed.* American Society for Surgery of the Hand. Amsterdam: Churchill Livingstone.

Pathways Awareness. (2011) *Tummy-time central.* Retrieved from http://www. pathwaysawareness.org/tummytime (Excellent website for parents and professionals. See links for research articles, brochures, and CMEs.)

Pendleton, H.M., & Schultz-Krohn, W. (Eds.) (2006). *Pedretti's occupational therapy practice skills for physical dysfunction.* St. Louis, MO: Mosby.

Peira, K., & Brown, A.J. (2008). Postpartum thyroiditis: Not just a worn out mother. *Journal for Nurse Practitioners*, 4(3), 175-182.

Pin, T., Eldridge, B., & Galea, M.P. (2007). A review of the effects of sleep position, play position, and equipment use on motor development in infants. *Developmental Medicine & Child Neurology*, 49, 858-867.

Sax, T.W., & Rosenbaum, R.B. (2006). Neuromuscular disorders in pregnancy. *Muscle & Nerve*, 34(5), 559-571.

Shaker, C.S. (2010). *NICU swallowing and feeding: In the nursery and after discharge.* Seminar sponsored by: Pediatric Resources Inc., California

Speicher, T., Martin, R.D., & DeSimone, R.M. (2006). Managing low back pain through activities-of-daily-living education. *Athletic Therapy Today*, 11(6), 74-77.

Waitzman, K.A. (2007). The importance of positioning the near-term infant for sleep, play, and development. *Newborn and Infant Nursing Reviews*, 7(2), 76-81.

Wiet, G.J., Sie, K., Biavati, M.J., & Rocha-Worley, G. (2010). *Cleft palate.* Retrieved from http://emedicine.medscape.com

Wolf, L.S., & Glass, R.P. (2011). *Feeding & swallowing disorders in infants: implications for breast- and bottle-feeding.* Seminar sponsored by Seattle Children's Hospital, Seattle, Washington, May 21-22.

Quick Health Data Online for Breastfeeding

Quick Health Data Online provides state- and county-level data for all 50 states, the District of Columbia, and U.S. territories and possessions. Data are available by gender, race, and ethnicity, and come from a variety of national and state sources. The system is organized into eleven main categories, including demographics, mortality, natality, reproductive health, violence, prevention, disease, and mental health. Within each main category, there are numerous subcategories.

Quick Health Data Online offers many different types of data related to Breastfeeding, Maternal Health and Reproductive Health including information on:

» Percent of children ever breastfed,
» Percent of children exclusively breastfed at 3 and 6 months, and,
» Percent of children breastfed at 6 and 12 months.

Data on the system are provided for men and women with race and ethnicity details to enable comparisons between different population groups. Data can be used to generate tables such as these, which presents the percentages of children breastfed ever, at 6 months and at 12 months and the percentages of children exclusively breastfed at 3 months and exclusively breastfed at 6 months.

USLCA

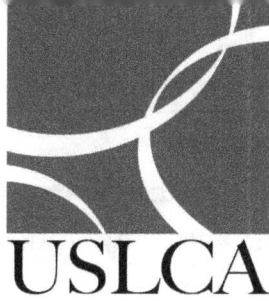

Breastfeeding and Dental Caries

Looking at the Evidence

Valerie Lavigne, DC, IBCLC, RLC[1]

Keywords: breastfeeding, dental caries, dental cavities, risk factors

Dental caries and prolonged breastfeeding still trigger much debate among professionals and parents. Some mothers are still being told to discontinue breastfeeding their toddlers because of cavities in the mouth. Parents often feel very discouraged and upset when they are forced to stop breastfeeding their toddlers. Dental caries is one of the most common chronic diseases in childhood, and is a disease of multifactorial etiology. This paper reviews the literature on dental caries and breastfeeding. This review revealed that there was no conclusive evidence that prolonged breastfeeding increased the risk of early childhood cavities.

Mothers around the globe are encouraged to breastfeed according to the recommendations of the World Health Organization, which states that babies should be

---

1   Valerielavigne@me.com

exclusively breastfed for the first six months, and up to two years and beyond with the addition of complementary food (World Health Organization, 2011). The Canadian Pediatric Society also endorses these recommendations. The health benefits of breastfeeding have been shown to reduce sudden infant death syndrome, otitis media, asthma, breast cancer, and accelerate postpartum weight loss. However, the American Academy of Pediatric Dentistry (AAPD) does not endorse the recommendation of extended breastfeeding past 12 months of age, or after the first tooth eruption, as they believe it poses a risk for early childhood cavities (ECC) (American Academy of Pediatrics Dentistry, 2011).

Dental caries is one of the most common chronic diseases in childhood, creating severe problems worldwide (Losso et al., 2009). In 2003, the AAPD defined ECC as the presence of one or more decayed (non-cavitated or cavitated), missing (due to caries), or filled tooth surfaces in any primary tooth in a child up to 71 months of age or younger (Iida et al., 2007; Losso et al., 2009; Prakash et al., 2012; Ribeiro & Ribeiro, 2004). The prevalence of ECC is thought to be five times higher than asthma, and seven times higher than allergic rhinitis, ranging from 1% to 12% in preschoolers of developed countries and from 50%-80% in high-risk groups (Prakash et al., 2012; Ribeiro & Ribeiro, 2004). Teeth play an important role in digestion of food, in keeping spacing for the secondary teeth, in helping with speech development and contributing to social skills and confidence (Valaitis et al., 2000). EEC, when left untreated, has been linked with pain, bacteremia, compromised chewing, toxic overdose of analgesics, followed by malocclusion in permanent dentition, phonetic problems, lower self-esteem, and failure to thrive (Azevedo et al., 2005; Prakash et al., 2012). Identifying the risk factors associated with ECC are very important to help prevent the condition, as children often require costly treatment with hospitalization under sedation or general anesthesia (Prakash et al., 2012). The estimation of cost to repair ECC ranges between $200 and $6000 if general anesthesia and hospitalization are required (Udin, 1999).

Causes of Early Childhood Caries

ECC is a disease of multifactorial etiology. The main factors are: a) cariogenic bacteria, b) fermentable carbohydrate diet, c) susceptible tooth and host, and d) time (Harris et al., 2004; Losso et al., 2009; Prakash et al., 2012). ECC has also been linked with the following risk factors: demographics characteristics, oral hygiene practice, parental attitudes, educational status of the mother, temperament of child, pacifiers dipped in honey, frequent medication, and feeding habits (Azevedo et al., 2005; Prakash et al., 2012). Another risk factor worth noting from some preliminary studies is the association between the maternal level of vitamin D during pregnancy and the impact on primary dentition and ECC. It showed that mothers of children with ECC had significantly lower levels of vitamin D (Schroth, 2010).

The cariogenic micro-organisms involved in ECC are the *Streptococcus Mutans* and *Streptococcus Sobrinus*

(Ribeiro & Ribeiro, 2004). The infection of *Streptococcus* is done by vertical transmission from the mother's saliva containing high levels of *Streptococcus* at a very specific time called "window of infectivity." The severity of ECC has been directly linked to the level of bacteria in the mouth and the early infection. The bacteria have been found to be present as early as 6 months of age, even before tooth eruption (Losso et al., 2009; Prakash et al., 2012). Caries start with the bacteria infection, which then accumulate and multiply on the teeth biofilm or hard surface. This, combined with the prolonged exposure to carbohydrate, allows for the fermentation of the sugar inside the dental plaque, causing enamel demineralization, resulting in cavities (Retnakumari & Cyriac, 2012; Ribeiro & Ribeiro, 2004; Udin, 1999).

There is an association between frequency of carbohydrate exposure and caries, and whether the contact occurs mainly between meals and during sleep. During these periods, the saliva decreases and does not flush the carbohydrate away from the teeth, therefore allowing the bacteria to ferment (Losso et al., 2009). Breast milk has been shown to have a higher level of carbohydrate, which could potentially make it more cariogenic (Erickson & Mazhari, 1999). However, the level of cariogenicity of breast milk has been studied and the results showed that breast milk alone, in an in-vitro model, was not cariogenic and did not cause plaque ph reduction and enamel decalcification. Breast milk combined with a sugar rich diet can allow for bacterial fermentation and can become cariogenic (Erickson & Mazhari, 1999). The diet and bacteria level, therefore, play an important role in the development of ECC.

As shown, this disease is multifactorial and controversial amongst different professional associations. This paper will then look at the evidence available in the literature to establish if there is an association between prolonged breastfeeding and ECC.

Method

To investigate this question, the Cochrane library was searched using the following terms: "breastfeeding and dental caries." A Randomized Control Trial (RCT) was found relevant to the topic (Kramer et al., 2007). PubMed was searched, using the following Mesh terms: "breastfeeding and dental caries." Limits were added for systematic reviews, which resulted in three relevant articles (Ribeiro & Ribeiro, 2004; Valaitis et al., 2000; White, 2008). Another limit was applied to look for RCT and resulted in the same study already found in Cochrane search. When removing the limits, the search produced 212 articles. Some of the relevant and available articles were included in the analysis. PubMed was searched again using other terms relevant to the topic "breastfeeding and dental cavities," and resulted in 285 articles. Some longitudinal and cohort studies were kept for analysis (Arora et al., 2011; Azevedo et al., 2005; Iida et al., 2007; Mohebbi et al., 2008; Prakash et al., 2012; Retnakumari & Cyriac, 2012; Tanaka & Miyake, 2012). Hand searching through the references of the articles was performed to locate other relevant information (Harris et al., 2004; Losso et al., 2009; Weerheijm et al., 1998).

Results

The search for the highest level of evidence on dental caries and prolonged breastfeeding revealed only one RCT (Kramer et al., 2007). The cluster RCT looked at the effect of an intervention to promote breastfeeding (Promotion of Breastfeeding Intervention Trial: PROBIT) in Belarus. Children were then followed up at 6.5 years of age to determine the effects on breastfeeding and dental caries. The study randomized maternity hospital units (clusters) and one affiliated polyclinic per hospital with double randomization based on both a random numbers table and a coin flip. The experiment implemented the Baby-Friendly Hospital Initiative in the clusters hospital, whereas the control hospital continued their normal practices and policies that were in effect.

The results are based on 17,046 healthy breastfed children from 31 maternity wards. The study results showed an increased rate of any breastfeeding at 3, 6, 9, and 12 months. The prevalence of exclusive breastfeeding was seven times higher in the PROBIT group versus the control. At 6.5 years of age, 81.5% of children had a dental examination follow-up. The dental examination data were recorded in the PROBIT data form. The results showed no significant difference in decayed, missing, or filled teeth (DMFT) between the experimental and control group. The total number of DMFT in the experimental group was 4.3 (3.7%) and in the control group, it was 4.2 (3.4%).

The authors then concluded that there is no reduction in caries risk with prolonged and exclusive breastfeeding. The authors addressed a limitation of their study being that routine examinations were performed by a large number of uncalibrated public health dentists. One weakness of the study is that by the age of dental evaluation being 6.5 years, some children may have lost a majority of their deciduous incisors teeth, which may have underestimated the effects. Another weakness to consider is that the study showed an increase in breastfeeding rate with the PROBIT, but the breastfeeding duration is not known for the children that developed caries. Nonetheless, this is a very interesting study due to the large sample size and the randomized experimental design.

Evidence from Systematic Reviews

The next level of evidence to consider was systematic reviews. White (2008) produced a systematic review to answer a clinical scenario using a PICO (populationin-tervention-comparison-outcome) style question: "Does continuation of breastfeeding increase the risk of early childhood caries in infants of over 6 months of age compared with other methods of infant feeding?" This was a well-performed review. The author described her search strategy and mesh terms used, and showed a table of summary of the relevant papers. Her review concluded that there is a lack of consistent evidence linking breastfeeding to the development of ECC. She suggests that an emphasis should be placed on promoting good oral hygiene practice from the time of eruption of the first tooth, and giving parents advice on reducing the frequency and consumption of sugar containing foods and drinks.

Another review by Ribeiro and Ribeiro (2004) looked at ECC and breastfeeding. The study described the ECC problem well, possible etiologies, and the role of breast milk. However, the review did not describe in detail the search strategy used to find the studies. The studies used were displayed in a table, but there were no details on the quality assessment process for the articles in the review. The studies were difficult to compare due to inconsistent results. However, they still were able to conclude that there were no scientific association between human milk and ECC. They do state that this is a complex relation to establish and that there are many variables that can affect the relationship.

Valaitis et al. (2000) produced another systematic review. This review followed a strong methodology, which is described step-by-step in a table. They offered a description of the ECC problem and showed a figure on the interrelationships of factors in the development of ECC. The review included 28 relevant articles, and the authors did assess the quality of the study. They mentioned that no articles of strong quality were included and only findings from articles rated as moderate and weak were presented. They noted that some of the results of the studies often contradict one another and findings are not always reproducible. However, they still concluded that the evidence does not suggest a consistent and strong association between breastfeeding and ECC. They do suggest that future research should be performed with more rigorous research methods.

Evidence from Cross-Sectional Studies

Some other studies of interest used retrospective cross-sectional data. Nunes et al. (2012) did a retrospective cohort study involving a sample size of 206 low-income children. This study had a clear description of the inclusion and exclusion criteria. They also used a seven-level hierarchical theoretical framework model to control for the variables associated with ECC. The results showed that prolonged breastfeeding was not a risk factor for ECC after adjusting for some confounders. Interestingly, they did state that age, high sucrose consumption between meals, and the quality of oral hygiene were associated with ECC.

Mohebbi (2008) performed a cross-sectional study with a sample size of 504 children. He concluded that milk bottle-feeding at night should be limited and was associated to ECC, whereas prolonged breastfeeding appears to have no such negative dental consequences. Another study (Iida et al. 2007) looked at a sample size of 1,576 children, aged two-to-five years old. The results of the different models used to analyze the data showed no evidence that either breastfeeding or its duration was independently associated with an increased risk of ECC. One weakness to note from a retrospective study is the data may be subject to recall bias. Also, in this study some of the confounding variables were not adjusted for due to lack of available data. However, this study is definitely worth noting, considering the large sample size.

Azevedo (2005), in contrast, showed a positive association between prolonged breastfeeding and ECC. One important element that was not taken at all into consideration, or adjusted for in this study, was the food habits, snacks between meals, which would have an impact on the results. Tanaka and Miyake (2012) showed that breastfeeding for 18 months or longer was positively associated with the prevalence of dental caries, whereas breastfeeding for 6 to 17 months was non-significantly inversely associated with the prevalence of dental caries. Their sample size was 2,056 children, aged 3 years old. The information was obtained by questionnaire, and the study did adjust for confounders. However, a major weakness is that the breastfeeding duration was the period during which the infants received breast milk, regardless of exclusivity. This poses a problem and may have contributed to dental caries if children were exposed to bottles and formula at any point. They do state that the study still may have many confounding factors that cannot be controlled, and therefore, no cause and effect relationship should be drawn.

Discussion

After completing this research, the most striking find is that ECC is a disease of multiple causes. It becomes difficult to isolate one element and a cause and effect when performing studies. When looking at ECC and breast-feeding alone, a link between the two has been difficult to establish. Some factors to consider that may have an effect are the level of bacteria present in the mouth, a suscep-tible host and a high sugar (sucrose) intake. Breast milk contains carbohydrates and sugar. However, it was only when mixed with other food that this became an issue. Breastfeeding children with higher levels of bacteria may have more ECC when compared to other breastfeeding children with lower levels of bacteria.

Some authors reported that *S. mutans* may not be able to use lactose, the sugar found in breast milk, as readily as sucrose, found in food or artificial milk, and some breast-milk antibodies may help impede bacterial growth (Mandel, 1996; Rugg-Gunn et al., 1985). One must remember that the bacteria were shown to be transferred from the mother at a specific time in the toddler's life.

It is also important to understand that the mechanics of breastfeeding versus bottle feeding are very different. When babies breastfeed, the nipple is drawn far back in the mouth and the milk is released into the throat more directly, whereas in bottle feeding, the milk pools around the teeth. The use of a bottle is associated with reduced salivary flow, which would cause the fermentable carbohydrate to pool around the teeth and promote the development of ECC (Ribeiro & Ribeiro, 2004).

In my opinion, the most important factor, which is common to many of these studies, that contributes to

ECC is the level of sugar-rich food and between-meal snacks that are consumed. This, combined with a high level of bacteria, seems to contribute to ECC. It is then crucial that parents be informed on proper dental hygiene for their children from infancy, and be sensitized towards the appropriate non-cariogenic snacks to feed them. Therefore, the mother's decision to continue breastfeeding should not be affected by the appearance of dental caries in their children, as no solid research has shown a direct link between the two.

Conclusion

Mothers should be encouraged to breastfeed as long as they desire, since no conclusive evidence has established a relationship between prolonged breastfeeding and the development of ECC.

References

American Academy of Pediatrics Dentistry. (2011). *Policy on Early Childhood Caries (ECC): Classifications, consequences, and preventive strategies.* Retrieved from: http://www.aapd.org/media/Policies_Guidelines/P_ECCClassifications.pdf

Arora, A., Scott, J.A., Bhole, S., Do, L., Schwarz, E., & Blinkhorn, A. S. (2011). Early childhood feeding practices and dental caries in preschool children: A multi-centre birth cohort study. *BMC Public Health, 11,* 28. doi: 10.1186/1471-2458-11-28

Azevedo, T. D., Bezerra, A. C., & de Toledo, O. A. (2005). Feeding habits and severe early childhood caries in Brazilian preschool children. *Pediatric Dentistry, 27*(1), 28-33.

Erickson, P.R., & Mazhari, E. (1999). Investigation of the role of human breast milk in caries development. *Pediatric Dentistry, 21*(2), 86-90.

Harris, R., Nicoll, A.D., Adair, P.M., & Pine, C. M. (2004). Risk factors for dental caries in young children: A systematic review of the literature. *Community Dental Health, 21*(1 Suppl), 71-85.

Iida, H., Auinger, P., Billings, R.J., & Weitzman, M. (2007). Association between infant breastfeeding and early childhood caries in the United States. *Pediatrics, 120*(4), e944-952. doi: 10.1542/peds.2006-0124

Kramer, M. S., Vanilovich, I., Matush, L., Bogdanovich, N., Zhang, X., Shishko, G., . . Platt, R.W. (2007). The effect of prolonged and exclusive breast-feeding on dental caries in early school-age children. New evidence from a large randomized trial. *Caries Research, 41*(6), 484-488. doi: 10.1159/000108596

Losso, E. M., Tavares, M. C., Silva, J. Y., & Urban Cde, A. (2009). Severe early childhood caries: An integral approach. *Journal of Pediatrics (Rio J), 85*(4), 295-300. doi: doi:10.2223/JPED.1908

Mandel, I. D. (1996). Caries prevention: Current strategies, new directions. *Journal of the American Dental Association, 127*(10), 1477-1488.

Mohebbi, S. Z., Virtanen, J. I., Vahid-Golpayegani, M., & Vehkalahti, M. M. (2008). Feeding habits as determinants of early childhood caries in a population where prolonged breastfeeding is the norm. *Community Dental and Oral Epidemiology, 36*(4), 363-369.

Nunes, A M., Alves, C.M., Borba de Araujo, F., Ortiz, T.M., Ribeiro, M.R., Silva, A. A., & Ribeiro, C.C. (2012). Association between prolonged breast-feeding and early childhood caries: A hierarchical approach. *Community Dental and Oral Epidemiology.* doi: 10.1111/j.1600-0528.2012.00703.x

Prakash, P., Subramaniam, P., Durgesh, B. H., & Konde, S. (2012). Prevalence of early childhood caries and associated risk factors in preschool children of urban Bangalore, India: A crosssectional study. *European Journal of Dentistry, 6*(2), 141-152.

Retnakumari, N., & Cyriac, G. (2012). Childhood caries as influenced by maternal and child characteristics in pre-school children of Kerala: An epidemiological study. *Contemporary Clinical Dentistry, 3*(1), 2-8. doi: 10.4103/0976-237x.94538

Ribeiro, N. M., & Ribeiro, M. A. (2004). Breastfeeding and early childhood caries: A critical review. *Journal of Pediatrics (Rio J), 80*(5 Suppl), S199-210.

Rugg-Gunn, A. J., Roberts, G.J., & Wright, W.G. (1985). Effect of human milk on plaque pH in situ and enamel dissolution in vitro compared with bovine milk, lactose, and sucrose. *Caries Research, 19*(4), 327-334.

Schroth, R. J. (2010). *Influence of maternal prenatal vitamin d status on infant oral health.* University of Manitoba. Retrieved from http://hdl.handle.net/1993/4274

Tanaka, K., & Miyake, Y. (2012). Association between breastfeeding and dental caries in Japanese children. *Journal of Epidemiology, 22*(1), 72-77.

Udin, R. D. (1999). Newer approaches to preventing dental caries in children. *Journal of the California Dental Association, 27*(11), 843-851.

Valaitis, R., Hesch, R., Passarelli, C., Sheehan, D., & Sinton, J. (2000). A systematic review of the relationship between breastfeeding and early childhood caries. *Canadian Journal of Public Health, 91*(6), 411-417.

Weerheijm, K. L., Uyttendaele-Speybrouck, B.F., Euwe, H.C., & Groen, H.J. (1998). Prolonged demand breast-feeding and nursing caries. *Caries Research, 32*(1), 46-50.

White, V. (2008). Breastfeeding and the risk of early childhood caries. *Evidence-Based Dentistry, 9*(3), 86-88. doi: 10.1038/sj.ebd.6400603

World Health Organization. (2011, January 15, 2011). *Exclusive breastfeeding for six months best for babies everywhere.* Retrieved from: http://www.who.int/mediacentre/news/ statements/2011/breastfeeding_20110115/en/

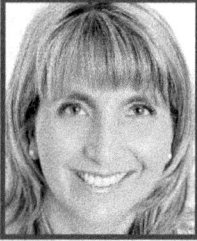

Valerie Lavigne, DC, IBCLC, RLC graduated from the Canadian Memorial Chiropractic College in 1998. In July 2005, she became an IBCLC, the first chiropractor in Quebec with the title. She has her fellowship in pediatrics from the International Chiropractic Pediatric Association and has started a Master of Science at the Anglo-European Chiropractic College in Pediatric musculoskeletal health. She is working as a chiropractor in her chiropractic clinic in Kirkland, Quebec and as an IBCLC at the Herzl Goldfarb Breastfeeding Clinic since 2010.

Guidelines for the Care of Late Preterm Infants

The U.S. National Perinatal Association has recently released Multidisciplinary Guidelines for the Care of Late Preterm Infants. The guidelines, developed by a multidisciplinary team initiated at a 2010 summit, give health care providers and others a roadmap to focus attention on the unique needs of late preterm infants, from birth through early childhood, helping to ensure potential health risks are not overlooked. This document outlines strategic approaches to evaluating and managing the care of late preterm infants for physicians, midwives, nurses, ancillary members of the health care team, and parents. Topics include in-hospital assessment and care, transition to outpatient care, short-term follow-up care, and long-term follow-up care.

Source: Coalition for Improved Maternity Services

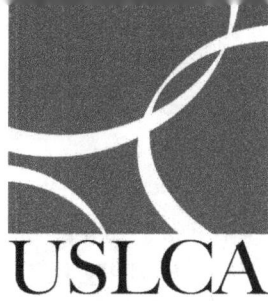

Pediatric Nurses' Knowledge and Attitudes Regarding the Provision of Breastfeeding Support in a Pediatric Medical Center

Tracy L. Brewer, DNP, RNC-OB, CLC[1]

Keywords: knowledge, attitudes, breastfeeding, support, pediatric nurses

Breastfeeding is the biological norm for infant feeding and nutrition. Successful breastfeeding depends, in part, on the support of the nursing staff caring for the breastfeeding dyad. Many infants are admitted to pediatric hospitals during the period when breastfeeding skills are being established, and mothers look to pediatric nurses to provide breastfeeding

1   Tracy.Brewer@Wright.edu

support and resources. There are few studies describing pediatric nurses' knowledge of and attitudes towards the provision of breastfeeding support in pediatric medical centers. The purpose of this descriptive survey study was to determine knowledge and attitudes of pediatric nurses regarding the provision of breastfeeding support. The Theory of Reasoned Action provided the framework for the study. A convenience sample of 92 pediatric nurses, on three inpatient units at a pediatric medical center, completed a 40-item breastfeeding survey. Seventy-seven complete surveys were returned for a usable response rate of 84%. Results indicated that pediatric nurses have moderate breastfeeding knowledge and attitudes. The pediatric nurses who had personal breast-feeding experience had significantly higher knowledge and attitude scores. Findings suggest the need for evidence-based educational programs to improve pediatric nurses' knowledge of and attitudes towards the provision of breastfeeding support in pediatric medical centers.

Breastfeeding is the biological norm for infant feeding and nutrition. It has been well documented that human milk is the preferred food for all infants, including premature and sick newborns (American Academy of Pediatrics [AAP], 2005). The World Health Organization (WHO) and the American Academy of Pediatrics (AAP) (2005) recommend that infants be exclusively breastfed without supplemental foods or liquids for the first 6 months of life (Kramer & Kakuma, 2007). Successful breastfeeding depends, in part, on the support of the nursing staff directly caring for the breastfeeding dyad.

Traditionally, it has been the role of obstetrical nurses to support mothers' initiation of breastfeeding. However, with early discharge from the hospital, many infants are admitted to pediatric facilities within the first 2 to 4 weeks of life with problems, such as dehydration, excessive weight loss, failure to thrive, or hyperbilirubinemia (Spatz & Goldschmidt, 2006; Tyler & Hellings, 2003). Frequently, these admissions are a direct result of a mother not fully understanding how to breastfeed her infant (Narramore, 2007). An infant's readmission to a pediatric medical facility should not be the cause of discontinuation of breastfeeding (Watkins & Dodgson, 2010). Breastfeeding duration has been recognized to decline after discharge from the birth hospital (Lawrence & Lawrence, 2008), with the most significant decline occurring within the first 2 weeks postpartum (Bernaix et al., 2010). Therefore, it becomes the role of the pediatric nurse to safeguard continuation and exclusivity of breastfeeding while the infant is admitted to a pediatric medical center.

Several factors can influence the initiation, duration, and exclusivity of successful breastfeeding including provision of accurate information and support to breast-feeding mothers by health care providers during the early weeks of breastfeeding establishment (Bernaix, 2000; Bernaix et al., 2010; Watkins & Dodgson, 2010). Inconsistent or inaccurate information and lack of support by health care professionals are reported factors affecting breastfeeding failure (Bernaix, 2000; Bernaix et al., 2010; Karipis & Spicer, 1999; Narramore, 2007; Spatz, 2010). Understanding what factors influences pediatric nurses' intent to provide breastfeeding support when infants are admitted to a pediatric hospital can be vital to the success (or failure) of a dyad's future breastfeeding experience. Several studies suggest that nurses' knowledge and attitudes predict their intention to provide breastfeeding support (Bernaix, 2000, Bernaix et al., 2010; Martens, 2000; Register et al., 2000; Siddell et al., 2003).

Additional research findings have proposed that nurses who have personal breastfeeding experience, or attain higher education, such as a bachelor's or graduate degree, are more likely to provide support and encouragement to breastfeeding dyads (Anderson & Geden, 1991; Barnett et al., 1995; Patton et al., 1996; Siddell et al., 2003). While most nurses receive some breastfeeding instruction in nursing school (Dodgson & Tarrant, 2007; Spear, 2006), few students have any clinical experience providing breastfeeding support. Mothers look to nurses as the "experts," yet pediatric nurses may only be able to rely on what they learned about breastfeeding during their nursing education, or through personal experience, as they provide breastfeeding support, which could result in inconsistent and/or inaccurate breastfeeding information.

However, little is known about pediatric nurses' knowledge of and attitudes towards breastfeeding and providing breastfeeding support in pediatric medical centers (Karipis & Spicer, 1999; Narramore, 2007), or the effectiveness of educational breastfeeding programs with this population of nurses. Therefore, it is first important to understand pediatric nurses' baseline knowledge and attitudes regarding the provision of breastfeeding support.

The purpose of this study was to determine knowledge and attitudes of pediatric nurses regarding the provision of support to breastfeeding dyads when the infant is admitted to a pediatric hospital. A second purpose explored the possible relationships between pediatric nurses' knowledge and attitudes toward providing breastfeeding support and select demographic variables, such as years of post-high school education and prior personal breastfeeding experience. The Theory of Reasoned Action provided the framework for the study.

Methods

Design and Setting

A descriptive-survey design was used to determine knowledge of and attitudes towards breastfeeding and breastfeeding support among a single sample of pediatric nurses. Institutional Review Board (IRB) approval was obtained from the study medical center. Participants were surveyed one time using a web-based survey. The setting for this study was a pediatric quaternary regional medical center in the Midwestern region of the United States.

Participants

A convenience sample of nurses was recruited from three inpatient units, which receive the largest proportion of breastfeeding-infant admissions. Each potential participant received an anonymous email invitation on the day the survey link became available, and a reminder email two weeks following the initial invitation. Consent was implied with the completion of the survey. Participants could withdraw from the study survey at any time.

Instruments

A 12–item demographic survey, originally developed by Siddell et al. (2003), was modified for the current study to investigate additional demographic items of age, ethnicity, and source of breastfeeding education. Original questions remained regarding personal breastfeeding experience, satisfaction with breastfeeding experience, years in current position, and years of post-high school education.

The Breastfeeding Survey is a 40-item question-naire developed for a study of neonatal nurses on the effectiveness of a breastfeeding educational intervention. The survey contains four subscales: knowledge regarding breastfeeding (KNOW) and three attitude scales; pro-breastfeeding attitudes (Pro-BF); attitudes representing baby-focused care (BFC); and attitudes representing nurse-focused care (NFC) (Siddell et al., 2003).

Responses to each of the items were on a five-point Likert scale from strongly disagree (1) to strongly agree (5). Responses from the KNOW subscale were summed for a total knowledge score ranging from 13 to 65. Responses to the three attitude subscales were combined into a one, 27-item subscale, and totaled for a single attitude score ranging from 27 to 135. The higher either subscale score, the greater the nurse's breastfeeding knowledge and positive attitude toward breastfeeding and providing breastfeeding support.

Previous content validity of the attitude and knowledge subscales was derived from a review of the breastfeeding attitudes and current breastfeeding practice trends literature (Siddell et al, 2003.). Reliability of the Breastfeeding Survey was established in the current study for internal consistency of the knowledge and attitude scales. The Cronbach's alpha for the knowledge and attitude scales were .66 and .69 respectively.

Results

The data were analyzed using the Statistical Package for the Social Sciences (SPSS). Ninety-two surveys were returned. However, two of the surveys were blank and 13 of the surveys had incomplete data. These surveys were removed from the data set and were not analyzed, leaving 77 completed surveys for a usable survey response rate of 84%.

Sample Characteristics

Participants' mean age was 31.6 years (SD = 8.7), ranging from 22 to 60 years of age. The participants had worked an average of 5.80 years (SD = 5.8), with a range of 1 to 30 years in their current position. Over half of the participants' (55%) highest degree in nursing was a bachelor's degree.

Nursing school was the primary source of breast-feeding information for a majority of the nurses (44.7%), though many also indicated they had learned about breastfeeding through hospital in-services (35.5%). Other sources of breastfeeding education included unit lactation consultants, nutritionists, and La Leche League. Almost half of the nurses (47.7%) participating in the study had personal breastfeeding experience. Of the 36 nurses who breastfed, 58.2% breastfed for over 6 months, and 80% stated they found breastfeeding a satisfying experience.

Pediatric Nurses Knowledge and Attitudes

Responses to the items on the knowledge scale and attitude scale were each individually summed for a total score. The mean knowledge score was 47.2 (SD = 5.1), and ranged from 32 to 61 out of a total possible score of 65. The mean attitude score was 91.9 (SD = 8.1), and ranged from 71 to 112 out of a possible total score of 135.

To assess the relationship between breastfeeding knowledge and years of education post high school, a Pearson-product moment correlation was calculated. No significant correlation was found between knowledge scores and years of post-high school education ($r = -.152$, $p = .189$). However, personal breastfeeding experience was significantly correlated with knowledge scores ($r = -.275$, $p = .025$). In addition, group differences were analyzed using an independent t-test to compare those nurses who had personal breastfeeding experience, and those nurses who had no personal breastfeeding experience, and their knowledge scores. Nurses who had a personal breast-feeding experience had significantly higher ($t(74) = 2.287$, p = .025) breastfeeding-knowledge scores than nurses who had no personal breastfeeding experience.

No significant correlation was found between attitude scores and years of education post-high school (r = -.142, p = .220), but attitude scores were significantly correlated with personal breastfeeding experience (r = -.259, p = .024). Attitude scores were analyzed for group differences using an independent t-test to compare those nurses who had personal breastfeeding experience and those nurses who had no personal breastfeeding experience. Nurses who had personal breastfeeding experience had significantly higher attitude scores than nurses who had no personal breastfeeding experience (t(74) = 2.306, p = .024).

Discussion

Pediatric nurses are frequently called upon to provide support and education to breastfeeding dyads when they are admitted to pediatric medical centers during the infant's first month of life, when breastfeeding is initially being established. However, it is suspected that pediatric nurses lack the knowledge and positive attitudes to provide adequate breastfeeding support to these breastfeeding dyads. Pediatric nurses participating in this study had only marginal knowledge and positive attitudes towards breastfeeding and breastfeeding support. Of concern is the finding that 44.7% of the nurses in this study indicated their primary source of breastfeeding knowledge was nursing school. If nursing school is a primary source of breastfeeding knowledge, then greater emphasis needs to be placed on breastfeeding education in schools of nursing, including specific breastfeeding education aimed at pediatric nurses (Watkins & Dodgson, 2010). In addition, since previous findings support that intent towards a behavior is influenced by positive attitudes, which may have predictive value towards nurses providing successful breastfeeding support (Bernaix, 2000; Bernaix et al., 2010; Siddell et al. 2003), one must be apprehensive that those nurses with poorer attitudes will resort to more deleterious behaviors towards the breastfeeding dyad.

Pediatric nurses in this study who had a personal breastfeeding experience had significantly higher breast-feeding knowledge and attitude scores than nurses who indicated they had no personal breastfeeding experience. One could possibly conclude that those nurses who had breastfed their own infants had a better understanding of, and confidence with, breastfeeding, and transferred that knowledge to their behaviors while supporting breast-feeding dyads at the bedside. In prior studies, a nurse's educational preparation was significantly correlated with breastfeeding knowledge and/or attitude scores among pediatric and obstetrical nurses (Patton et al., 1996; Siddell et al., 2003). No such relationship was found in the current study. This could be due to the fact that nearly 60% of the nurses already had a bachelors, or higher degree in nursing, indicating that this population of pediatric nurses already had higher level of nursing knowledge.

Limitations

Limitations for this study include a convenience sample of pre-selected nurses, a small number of participants primarily from one ethnic background, and only one sample from one geographic region. The findings, therefore, cannot be generalized to all pediatric-nursing populations. The convenience sample consisted of pediatric nurses' from only three select inpatient units at the pediatric medical center. The group was homogeneous, with 95% of the nurses being Caucasian and all being women. Of note, nearly 50% of nurses who did complete the survey had a personal breastfeeding experience, and of those with a breastfeeding experience, 80% reported the experience as positive. These findings may have influenced or biased these nurses towards completing the survey. Finally, internal consistency of the Breastfeeding Survey instrument was marginal.

Implications for Nursing Practice and Future Education

Pediatric nurses have been overlooked as providers that require positive attitudes and knowledge in which to provide breastfeeding support to mother/infant dyads. American mothers are still far from meeting the *Healthy People 2020* goals for the duration and exclusivity of breast-feeding (U.S. Department of Health & Human Services, 2011). The current study adds to the body of evidence that, like obstetrical nurses, pediatric nurses lack the knowledge, and/or have marginal attitudes to provide breastfeeding support to mother/infant dyads in pediatric medical centers.

Given the significance of nurses' supportive role in the establishment of breastfeeding, and the new understanding that pediatric nurses lack knowledge of and positive attitudes towards breastfeeding, I hope that nursing schools and pediatric medical centers will develop breastfeeding education programs for their students and staff. These educational programs need to exemplify the evidence-based practices of the *Ten Steps to Successful Breastfeeding for Hospitals*, as outlined by UNICEF/WHO from the Baby-Friendly Hospital™ Initiative (Baby-Friendly USA, 2010). Nevertheless, future research is needed to assess the effectiveness of educational interventions for pediatric nurses as an initial step toward nurses' knowledge base.

References

American Academy of Pediatrics [AAP]. (2005). Policy statement: Breastfeeding and the use of human milk. *Pediatrics, 115*, 496506. doi: 10.1542/peds.100.6.1035

Anderson, E., & Geden, E. (1990). Nurses' knowledge of breastfeeding. *JOGNN, 20*(1), 58-64.

Barnett, E., Sienkiewicz, M., & Roholt, S. (1995). Beliefs about breastfeeding: A statewide survey of health professionals. *Birth, 22*(1), 15-20.

Baby-Friendly USA, Inc. (2010). *Implementing the UNICEF/WHO Baby Friendly Hospital Initiative in the U.S.* Retrieved from http://www.babyfriendlyusa.org/eng/index.html

Bernaix, L.W. (2000). Nurses' attitudes, subjective norms, and behavioral intentions toward support of breastfeeding mothers. *Journal of Human Lactation, 16*(3), 201-208.

Bernaix, L.W., Beaman, M.L., Schmidt, C.A., Komives-Harris, J., & Mitchell-Miller, L. (2010). Success of an educational intervention on maternal/newborn nurses' breastfeeding knowledge and attitudes. *JOGNN, 39*, 658-666. doi: 10.1111/j.1552-6909.2010.01184.x

Dodgson, J.E., & Tarrant, M. (2007). Outcomes of a breastfeeding educational intervention for baccalaureate nursing students. *Nurse Education Today, 27*(8), 856-867. doi: 10.1016/j.nedt.2006.12.0001

Karipis, T. A., & Spicer, M. (1999). A survey of pediatric nurses' knowledge about breastfeeding. *Journal of Pediatric Nursing, 14*(3), 193-200.

Kramer, M.S., & Kakuma R. (2007). Optimal duration of exclusive breastfeeding. *Cochrane Database of Systematic Reviews, 4,* 1-2.

Lawrence, R.A., & Lawrence, R.M. (2008). *Breastfeeding: A guide for the medical profession.* St. Louis: Mosby.

Martens, P.J. (2000). Does breastfeeding education affect nursing staff beliefs, exclusive breastfeeding rates, and Baby-Friendly Hospital Initiative compliance? The experience of a small, rural Canadian hospital. *Journal of Human Lactation, 16*(4), 309-318.

Narramore, N. (2007). Supporting breastfeeding mothers on children's wards: An overview. *Paediatric Nursing, 19*(1), 18-21.

Patton, C.B., Beaman, M., Csar, N., & Lewinski, C. (1996). Nurses' attitudes and behaviors that promote breastfeeding. *Journal of Human Lactation, 12*(2), 111-115.

Register, N., Eren, M., Lowdermilk, D., Hammond, R., & Tully, M.R. (2000). Knowledge and attitudes of pediatric office nursing staff about breastfeeding. *Journal of Human Lactation, 16*(3), 210-215.

Siddell, E., Marnellie, K., Froman, R.D., & Burke, G. (2003). Evaluation of an educational intervention on breastfeeding for NICU nurses. *Journal of Human Lactation, 19*(3), 293-302. doi: 10.1177/0890334403255223

Spatz, D.L. (2010). The critical role of nurses in lactation support. *JOGNN, 39,* 499-500. doi: 10.1111/j.1552-6909.2010.01166.x

Spatz, D.L., & Goldschmidt, K.A. (2006). Preserving breastfeeding for the rehospitalized infant: A clinical pathway. *MCN, 31*(1), 45-51.

Spear, H.J. (2006). Baccalaureate nursing students' breastfeeding knowledge: A descriptive survey. *Nurse Education Today, 26,* 332337. doi: 10.1016/j.nedt.2005.10.014

Tyler, M., & Hellings, P. (2003). Feeding method and rehospitalization in newborns less than 1 month of age. *JOGNN, 34*(1), 70-79. doi: 10.1177/0884217504272813

U.S. Department of Health and Human Services (2011). *Healthy People 2020 Objectives: Maternal, infant, and child health.* Retrieved from http://www.healthypeople.gov/2020/ topicsobjectives2020/ objectiveslist.aspx?topicid=26

Watkins, A.L., & Dodgson, J.E. (2010). Breastfeeding educational interventions for health professionals: A synthesis of intervention studies. *Journal for Specialists in Pediatric Nursing, 15*(3), 223-232. doi: 10.1111/j.1744-6155.2010.00240.x

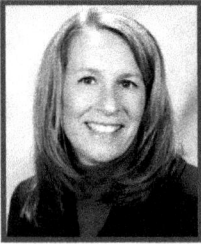

Dr. Tracy L. Brewer is an Assistant Professor at Wright State University, Miami Valley-College of Nursing and Health. In addition, Dr. Brewer is a certified lactation counselor and certified inpatient obstetrical nurse, with over 20 years experience working with mothers and babies. Dr. Brewer's current work is regarding the relationship between the dose of early hospital skin-to-skin contact and exclusivity of breast-feeding at 1 and 2 months of age.

USLCA

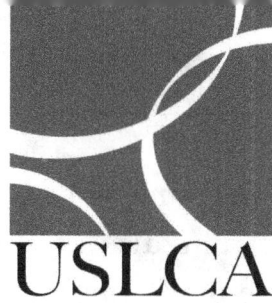

Supporting Breastfeeding Among Women on the Autistic Spectrum

Disability, Difference, and Delight

Dori Pelz-Sherman, PhD, CST[1]

Keywords: breastfeeding, Asperger's, high-functioning autism, disability, attachment, comorbid mood disorders with ASD

Professionals supporting breastfeeding mothers who are on the autistic spectrum by providing information, guidance, and clinical considerations for lactation in settings that are medical, psychological, or private practice in lactation support, may benefit from this comprehensive overview. The author outlines relevant symptoms and discusses how the practitioner-patient relationship could be impacted by characteristics associated with high-functioning autism and Asperger's, and includes a case study interview with a mother who has Asperger's. Practical guidelines for lactation support are included.

1   http://www.drpelz-sherman.com; dori@pelz-sherman.net

In recent decades, the number of individuals diagnosed with autistic spectrum disorders (ASDs) has risen significantly, yet the proportional dominance of males diagnosed (estimated 80% males) has resulted in a potentially underrecognized and underserved group of women with autism/Asperger's syndrome (AS), many of whom are becoming mothers and choosing to breastfeed. As this growing population enters obstetrical care, those diagnosed (and those who exhibit ASD characteristics but may not have received a formal diagnosis, meet the criteria, or have not disclosed their diagnosis) could benefit from care providers who have knowledge of and sensitivity to their specific lactation support needs. Women with autism have a variety of medical and behavioral considerations that endow them with vital implications for their physical and psychological well-being through the childbearing process (Bloch, Lecks, & Suplee, 2012). The objective of this article is to provide those who support mothers on the autistic spectrum with information, guidance, and clinical considerations for breastfeeding in settings that are medical, psychological, or private practice in lactation support.

Labels, Diagnosis, and Guidelines for Consideration

ASDs include high-functioning autism (HFA, common in the literature, but not a *Diagnostic and Statistical Manual of Mental Disorders, 5th Edition* [DSM-5] category) and AS. Although no longer included as a separate category in the

DSM-5, the classification of AS will be appropriated here to reflect the language that mothers may use to describe themselves, as well as to include a term that may be part of a medical record. For both AS and HFA, it is important to note that by definition, these terms are used when the individual's cognitive abilities measure as average or often above average. Deficits or differences are observed in behavior, communications, and often in sensory integration, and these are understood to be biologically based. Given the particular constellation of traits associated with spectrum disorders, these individuals may find personal relationships challenging (National Institute of Neurological Disorders and Strokes, 2005).

It is important to clarify that autism is not a childhood disorder; autism is a developmental disorder that will manifest differently throughout the lifespan; however, it is frequently first observed during childhood. Autism affects development and development affects autism (Frith, 2003). ASD is a neurodevelopmental disorder that may specifically affect use of language and cognitive styles, social acumen and interaction, sensory integration, flexibility, and interpersonal skills (Attwood, 2007; Frith, 2003). Each of these domains will be examined for their potential to impact breastfeeding; see "Guidelines for Consideration."

Diagnosis of AS/HFA is complex, and girls are further disadvantaged in part because traits associated with ASD exhibited in the manner observed with autism in early childhood, such as verbal expression, memory, and intelligence might not be as unusual for very young girls compared to the very young boys who are frequently expected to be much more active (Giarelli et al. 2010). Women frequently are diagnosed with AS later in life, unlike males; therefore, this population may not have benefited from either early intervention or social skill training, which has become increasingly available to boys and young men. Young women may have struggled with some social isolation, or others may have demonstrated a preference for what is referred to as social isolation. Some of these women, who may have a sense that they are socially "different," and recognize that they have difficulty understanding other people, may have negative expectancies about interpersonal relationships that have the potential for interfering with the mother–baby relationship. Interpersonal expectancies have been implicated in postpartum depression, which affects 15%-25% of childbearing women (Thompson & Bendell, in press).

For lactation consultants, the implications of these deficits or differences may mean that there is a need to reevaluate how to "read," and make meaning of, the observable behaviors of these new mothers. For example, a lack of eye contact may not mean disinterest, distrust, or non-genuine participation, but rather simply be the norm for the individuals' personal style and comfort in communication. With mindful attention to one's own inferences, the lactation instructor can accommodate the possible characteristics associated with autism with careful consideration.

Guidelines for Consideration

Certain characteristics that may be observed include awkward responses in normal social situations, frustration in interpreting social cues, inflexible routines or practices, being insensitive, or being less tuned into the emotions of those around them (National Institute of Neurological Disorders and Strokes, 2005). For lactation supporters, awareness of these possible characteristics increases the likelihood for possible modification of methods. These are general guidelines to assist professionals in developing or modifying their practice style. As with all autism treatments and accommodations, a subset of these will be applicable and effective with a subset of your mothers. Expect diversity.

» Use visual instructions, such as diagrams, outlines, or written instructions.

» For certain new mothers, it may be useful to adopt an uncharacteristically direct approach in your own verbal communication.

» Reduce the use of metaphors and rely more on concrete or literal language rather than abstract language.

» Avoid social innuendoes.

» Provide as much continuity of care (same person) such that the mother is not restarting a relationship repeatedly (if you are in a group practice).

» Be cautious in recommending groups, such as breastfeeding support groups in the community; individual support may better meet the mother's needs.

» Adopt a sensory sensitivity: consider the sounds, lighting, smells, and human stimulation in your working environment or in the home (e.g., if your office uses florescent lights, consider sky panels to diffuse the stimulation).

» Involve the mother's partner; that individual may have a way of "translating" information to her or to you that may be useful to your therapeutic relationship (while providing privacy).

» Be alert to guarding your own reactions against taking offense.

» Verbalize your intent to touch if there is physical contact on the course of your treatment; check in frequently in regard to touch and physical contact.

» Solicit questions; check for full understanding of your response.

» Consider reluctance to a suggestion you may make as possibly temporary; supplement with factual information and a well-supported rationale for your teaching.

» Listen for concrete speech and ask if you are unclear of her meaning.

» For some mothers, it may be useful to help her focus on measuring success on an individual basis—as opposed to what she may have read, even from a credible source. Professionals will be better able to meet the unique needs of women on the spectrum through consideration of the selected traits and examining how these might impact breastfeeding. However, it is equally important to remain cognizant that there is as much diversity of personality among individuals with AS because there is personality diversity among the neuro-typical (NT) population (Attwood, 2007). Traits and symptom constellations presented here may, at first glance, appear to have minor or moderate implications for impacting breastfeeding; however, it is critical to become aware that for an individual on the spectrum, a physical response can be experienced as extreme and debilitating, relative to the degree of discomfort, annoyance, or pain that an NT person (or person without autism) might report having experienced as a response to the same stimuli.

This is true for the woman's body as well; pain sensitivities may be hypersensitive or hyposensitive. For the lactation specialist, for example, this may mean not relying exclusively on verbal comfort or pain level reporting while supplementing through careful visual inspection and closely observing what you can see.

Difficulties in Recognizing Comorbid Autistic Spectrum Disorder and Mood Disorders

It is widely known that depression and the effects of mood disorders have a devastating impact on breastfeeding (Kendall-Tackett, 2010). We can surmise that would be true for women on the spectrum, but can only speculate as to the observable markers. Depression, like autism, is a diagnosis particularly constructed on a social framework; yet, although many studies exist for NT women, the studies for women on the spectrum with postpartum mood disorders have not been done. The social construction of depression has contributed to the reluctance to diagnose comorbid depression with autism (Ghaziuddin, 2005).

Attwood (2007) states that adults may be predisposed to depression in adulthood because of the cognitive style that is common in those with autism, along with feelings of alienation, mental fatigue from social efforts associated with their disability, and the culmination of a lifetime of social torment. It is possible that because the current clinical understanding of both conditions is limited by the DSM-5, the field of psychology, with some exceptions, has not recognized depression as a disorder among individuals with autism. Research has not yet produced a substantive description of the effects of depression in individuals with autism, nor specifically women with autism, and certainly not postpartum women. The debilitating effects of depression may further disadvantage women with ASD who already face significant social challenges that may negatively impact the transition to motherhood, and possibly impact breast-feeding and the parent-infant relationship.

Many autism specialists tend to overlook the signs and symptoms, and underdiagnose depression within the autism population (Ghaziuddin, Ghaziuddin, & Greden, 2002). The underdiagnosis of depression among people with autism could occur because practitioners may possibly attribute symptoms of depression to the primary diagnosis of autism, or underdiagnosis may be attributable to the phenomenon that the expression of symptoms of depression in people with autism does not fit preconceptions held by others regarding what depression might look like in an individual with autism. Alternatively, the person with autism may not be recognized to have enough social desire to experience social isolation associated with depression (Ghaziuddin, 2005).

Case Study Interview

In *The Autistic Brain*, Grandin (2013) writes about the shift away from a deficit model and toward a difference model; this is aptly illustrated by the reflections on breastfeeding that were offered by a mother with ASD. "Helene," a professional woman who had been diagnosed with AS and is currently living in the northeastern part of the U.S., agreed to be interviewed for the purpose of this article. She described having successfully nursed two babies born approximately 20 months apart. Helene describes remembering that she simply wanted the facts;

she wanted to know the science, and she wanted the data and the "how to." She had been advised to go to a La Leche League (LLL) meeting, and she describes the experience as having been somewhat helpful but that she knew she would not be returning. "Groups like that are not my thing; people were sort of flipping out and going over all their problems—but their [LLL] materials were really good." In addition, one phone call to a leader provided her with just the right information to get past the trouble she was experiencing at that time.

Helene describes that when she got the factual information, it was very useful to her. Initially, she reports that she did not know that "there were places where you're not supposed to nurse a baby, like church. I thought, if anyone had a problem with me feeding my baby, it was their problem and not my problem." With enthusiasm, she went on to explain, "I nursed on demand, anywhere, anytime. I was, and am, enormously attached to my boys. Babies are real. I'd rather spend time with a baby than go to a faculty meeting."

Helene had a good experience obtaining information to support her as a breastfeeding mother right from the beginning. When after pumping with no result, she was simply and directly told to just keep doing it anyway. She followed that advice, achieved a good outcome, and described the process of obtaining the support as useful and a good experience. In regard to the social factors, Helene reports, "If there was disapproval from anyone, I either would not have noticed or cared, because people have been disapproving of me since I was about 8. About the breastfeeding, I loved it."

There is a range in both number of characteristics of people with autism exhibited, as well as the degree to which each mother with autism is affected. When asked, Helene endorsed the guidelines provided here, and she suggested including the caveat that not everyone on the spectrum has sensory issues. The dominant social paradigm infers and supports the maxim that difference equates to lesser; that is, a reduced or diminished theory of mind. Molloy and Vasil (2002) give a strong voice to the difference versus disorder debate by pointing out that alternative conceptualizations have been absent in research and society, resulting in definitions being set by those with social and political power.

Being on the autistic spectrum will not necessarily disadvantage a mother in learning to breastfeed. However, because frequently, breastfeeding education and support are experienced in the context of a one-on-one helping relationship, the characteristics of AS/ASD/HFA may interfere if not considered and accommodated by the educator. For the lactation specialist, these factors may impact the helping relationship between the professional and the mother—a relationship that often exists on a continuum of apprenticeship, intimacy, and trust. Support may be more effective for the lactation consultant who applies mindful attention to adopting a flexible style of teaching—and when needed—a loosening of conventional rubrics regarding interpreting the mother's behavior and conceptualizing her struggles.

A genuine disinterest in the perceived judgments of others could work in a new mother's favor as she struggles to remain focused on her baby, on learning to breastfeed, and on negotiating the changes in her relationships with others. For the high-functioning woman with ASD, who is secure with herself, one might go so far as to wonder if AS could function as a benefit to the nursing mother.

In Closing

Lactation professionals are already highly skilled in customizing their approach to meet the needs of breast-feeding mothers because no two mothers and no two babies are alike. However, there are patterns of clinical need that can be considered and methods implemented to inform the specialist as she synthesizes the myriad of needs, attributions, and possibilities while supporting the mother-baby breastfeeding relationship experienced by mothers with ASD. Women with autism know they are not like other people in many ways and may offer profes-sionals the guidance needed to individualize the approach to care for those who can remain open, and can listen and learn. Although, when compared with the norms of dominant culture, there are distinct interaction patterns and preferences and cognitive and social differences; not all of these characteristics necessarily create impediments to breastfeeding nor is a social deficit necessarily an impediment to working well with lactation specialists.

Ortiz (2005) has championed the genuine qualities and positive gifts of refreshingly direct and honest communications and approach to relationships that individuals with AS contribute. Some people with ASD and HFA have spoken out publicly about their differences; however, specialists will need to approach such material with caution because, unlike other disabilities, autism and AS have attracted several self-diagnosed "spokespersons" who may or may not have information that is accurate or credible—posted or published by persons who, in fact, may not actually meet the medical and psychological criteria for autism. Some experts describe individuals on the spectrum as being easy targets and naive. For those who that aptly applies, support will be needed to guide mothers to credible information sources, and quality support. Mothers on the spectrum are likely to teach professionals a great deal about direct communication, speaking the truth, and difference, and may offer extremely enriching experiences.

References

Attwood, T. (2007). *The complete guide to Asperger's syndrome.* Philadelphia, PA: Jessica Kingsley.

Bloch, J. R., Lecks, K., & Suplee, P. D. (2012). Caring for women with Asperger's syndrome during the childbearing cycle. In E. Giarelli, & M. Gardner (Eds.), *Nursing of autism spectrum disorder: Evidence-based integrated care across the lifespan* (pp. 265–288). New York, NY: Springer Publishing.

Frith, U. (2003). *Autism, explaining the enigma* (2nd ed.). Oxford, United Kingdom: Blackwell.

Ghaziuddin, M. (2005). *Mental health aspects of autism and Asperger syndrome.* London, United Kingdom: Jessica Kingsley Publishers.

Ghaziuddin, M., Ghaziuddin, N., & Greden, J. (2002). Depression in persons with autism: Implications for research and clinical care. *Journal of Autism and Developmental Disorders, 32*(4), 299–306.

Giarelli, E., Wiggins, L. D., Rice, C. E., Levy, S. E., Kirby, R. S., Pinto-Martin, J., & Mandell, D. (2010). Sex difference in the evaluation and diagnosis of autistic spectrum disorders among children. *Disabilities Health Journal, 3*(2), 107–116.

Grandin, T. (2013). *The autistic brain: Thinking across the spectrum.* Boston, MA: Houghton Mifflin Harcourt.

Kendall-Tackett, K. A. (2010). *Depression in new mothers: Causes, consequences, and treatment alternatives (2nd ed.).* London, United Kingdom: Routledge.

Molloy, H., & Vasil, L. (2002). The social construction of Asperger syndrome: The pathologizing of difference. *Disability and Society, 17*(6), 659–669.

National Institute of Neurological Disorders and Strokes. (2013). *Asperger syndrome information page.* Retrieved from http://www.ninds.nih.gov/disorders/asperger/detail_asperger.htm

Ortiz, J. M. (2005). *The myriad gifts of Asperger's syndrome.* London, United Kingdom: Jessica Kingsley Publishers.

Thompson, K., & Bendell, D. (2014). Depressive cognitions, maternal attitudes, and postnatal depression. *Journal of Reproductive and Infant Psychology, 32*(1).

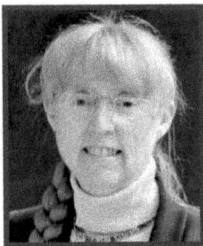

Dr. Dori Pelz-Sherman is a clinical psychologist, with a subspecialization in parent-infant mental health, and is currently in private practice in Raleigh, North Carolina. She is a medical advisor for Postpartum Education and Support (http://pesnc.org), and a former La Leche League leader and trainer. Selected publications include "Special Difficulties of Autism Spectrum Disorders in the Forensic Arena" in the *Handbook of Forensic Neuropsychology*, "Assessments" in *Autism: Asserting Your Child's Right to a Special Education*, and *Well-Being and Mitigating Factors for Depression Among Adolescents With High-Functioning Autism and Asperger's Syndrome*. Her website can be found at http://www.drpelz-sherman.com/

Fifth Circuit Holds Lactation Discrimination Is Unlawful Sex Discrimination

Overturning a federal trial court's decision from the Southern District of Texas, the U.S. Court of Appeals for the Fifth Circuit held unanimously that firing a woman because she is lactating or expressing milk is unlawful sex discrimination under Title VII of the Civil Rights Act of 1964 (as amended by the Pregnancy Discrimination Act of 1978). The appeal arose from a lawsuit filed by the Equal Employment Opportunity Commission (EEOC) on behalf of Donnica Venters, who claimed that she was fired after giving birth once she inquired as to whether she would be able to pump breast milk when she returned to her job. The EEOC sued, alleging that the employer, Houston Funding II, LLC, engaged in sex discrimination. The district court dismissed the lawsuit on a motion for summary judgment. Following that decision, the EEOC appealed to the Fifth Circuit. *Source: US Breastfeeding Committee*

Department of Health and Human Services' Infant Mortality Report

The Report of the Secretary's Advisory Committee on Infant Mortality (SACIM): Recommendations for Department of Health and Human Services Action and Framework for a National Strategy provides a plan to reduce infant mortality in the United States. The report includes an outline of strategic directions and recommendations, background on the problem, principles for a national strategy, and details related to six strategic directions for reducing infant mortality. Also discussed is information on services to improve women's health, birth outcomes, infant health, and infant survival; opportunities to decrease infant mortality through implementation of the Affordable Care Act; a crosswalk between an action plan to reduce racial and ethnic health disparities and recommendations to reduce infant mortality; and specific actions to increase breastfeeding. *Source: US Breastfeeding Committee*

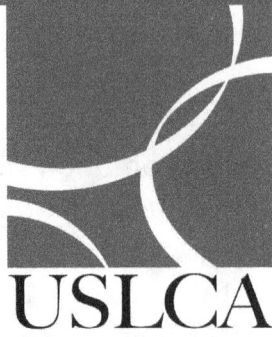

USLCA is a non-profit membership association focused on advancing the International Board Certified Lactation Consultant (IBCLC) in the United States through leadership, advocacy, professional development, and research.

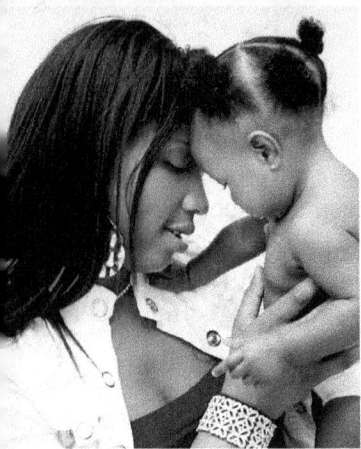

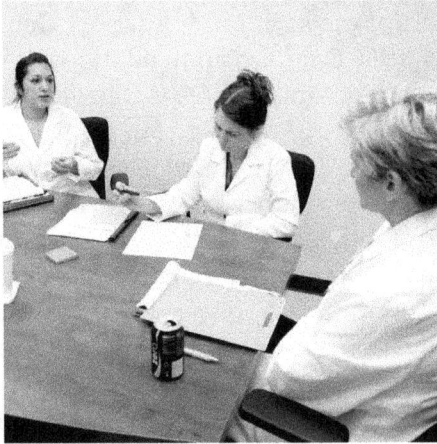

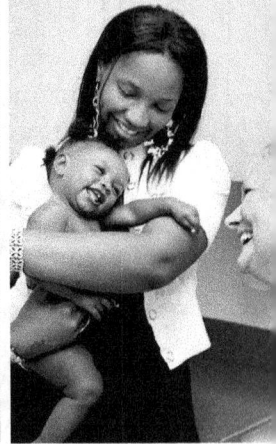

Join USLCA today
202-738-1125 | Washington, D.C. | www.USLCA.org

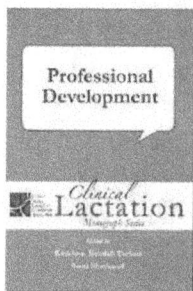

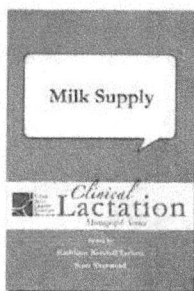

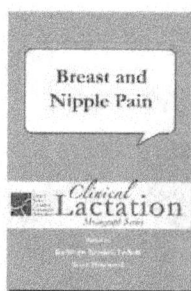

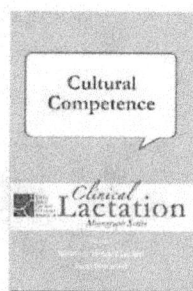

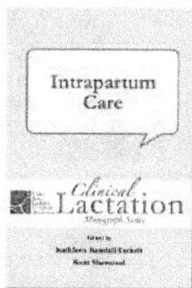

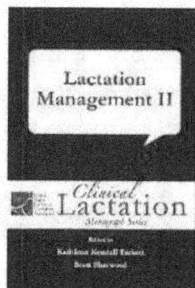

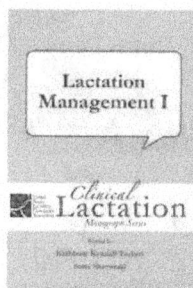

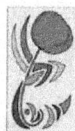

Breastfeeding and Women's Health Titles from Praeclarus Press

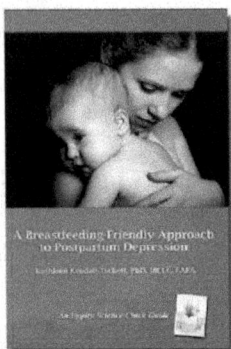

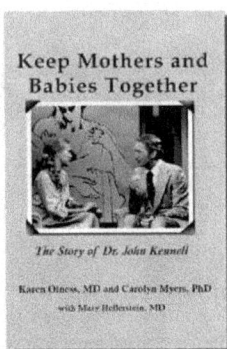

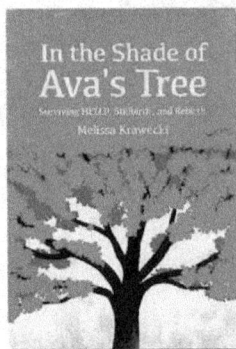

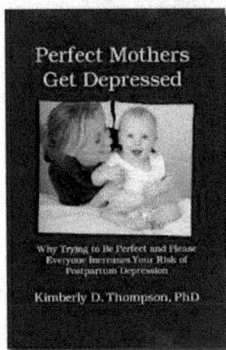

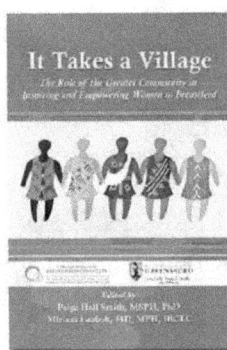

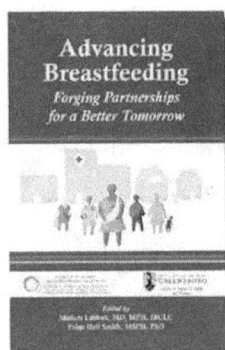

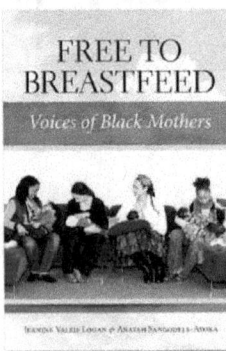

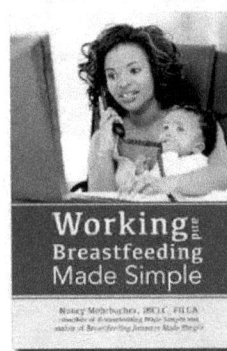

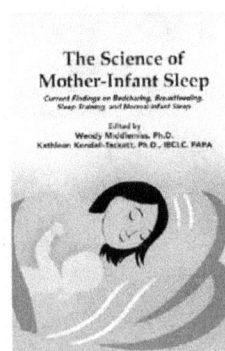

A Breastfeeding-Friendly Approach to Postpartum Depression

An Equity Wellness Chick Guide

Kathleen Kendall-Tackett, PhD, IBCLC, FAPA

Keep Mothers and Babies Together

The Story of Dr. John Kennell

Karen Olness, MD and Carolyn Myers, PhD
with Mary Hellerstein, MD

In the Shade of Ava's Tree

Surviving HELLP, Stillbirth, and Rebirth

Melissa Krawecki

Perfect Mothers Get Depressed

Why Trying to Be Perfect and Please Everyone Increases Your Risk of Postpartum Depression

Kimberly D. Thompson, PhD

It Takes a Village

The Role of the Greater Community in Inspiring and Empowering Women to Breastfeed

Edited by
Paige Hall Smith, MSPH, PhD
Miriam Labbok, MD, MPH, IBCLC

Advancing Breastfeeding

Forging Partnerships for a Better Tomorrow

Edited by
Miriam Labbok, MD, MPH, IBCLC
Paige Hall Smith, MSPH, PhD

FREE TO BREASTFEED

Voices of Black Mothers

JEANINE VALRIE LOGAN & ANAYAH SANGODELE-AYOKA

Working and Breastfeeding Made Simple

Nancy Mohrbacher, IBCLC, FILCA

The Science of Mother-Infant Sleep

Current Findings on Bedsharing, Breastfeeding, Sleep Training, and Normal Infant Sleep

Edited by
Wendy Middlemiss, Ph.D.
Kathleen Kendall-Tackett, Ph.D., IBCLC, FAPA

Praeclarus Press
Excellence in Women's Health

www.PraeclarusPress.com

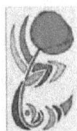